This book belongs

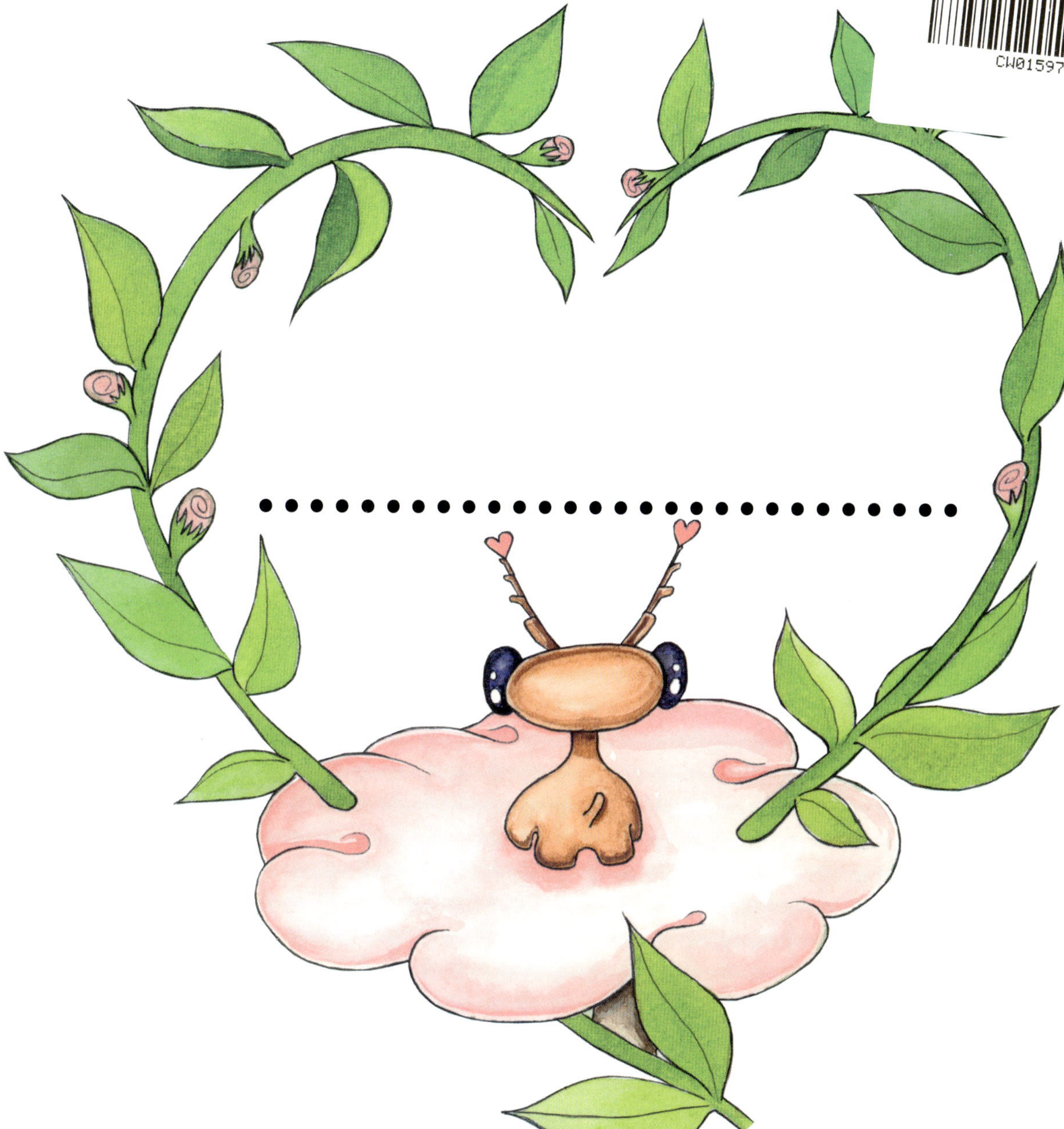

....

For Jasmine and Casper my little buds of inspiration, Carolyne for her encouragement at Horse World, Mum and Dad for everything and Richard for everything else. - J.G.

For Ruby, Felix and Pete, the most enchanting beings I know - S.O.

The Enchanted Child

First published in 2014 by Awespace
35 Carlton Street
Old Trafford
Manchester M16 7QU
www.awespace.org
ISBN: 978-0-9929095-0-5

Printed in Oxford by Berforts Information Press

The Enchanted Child

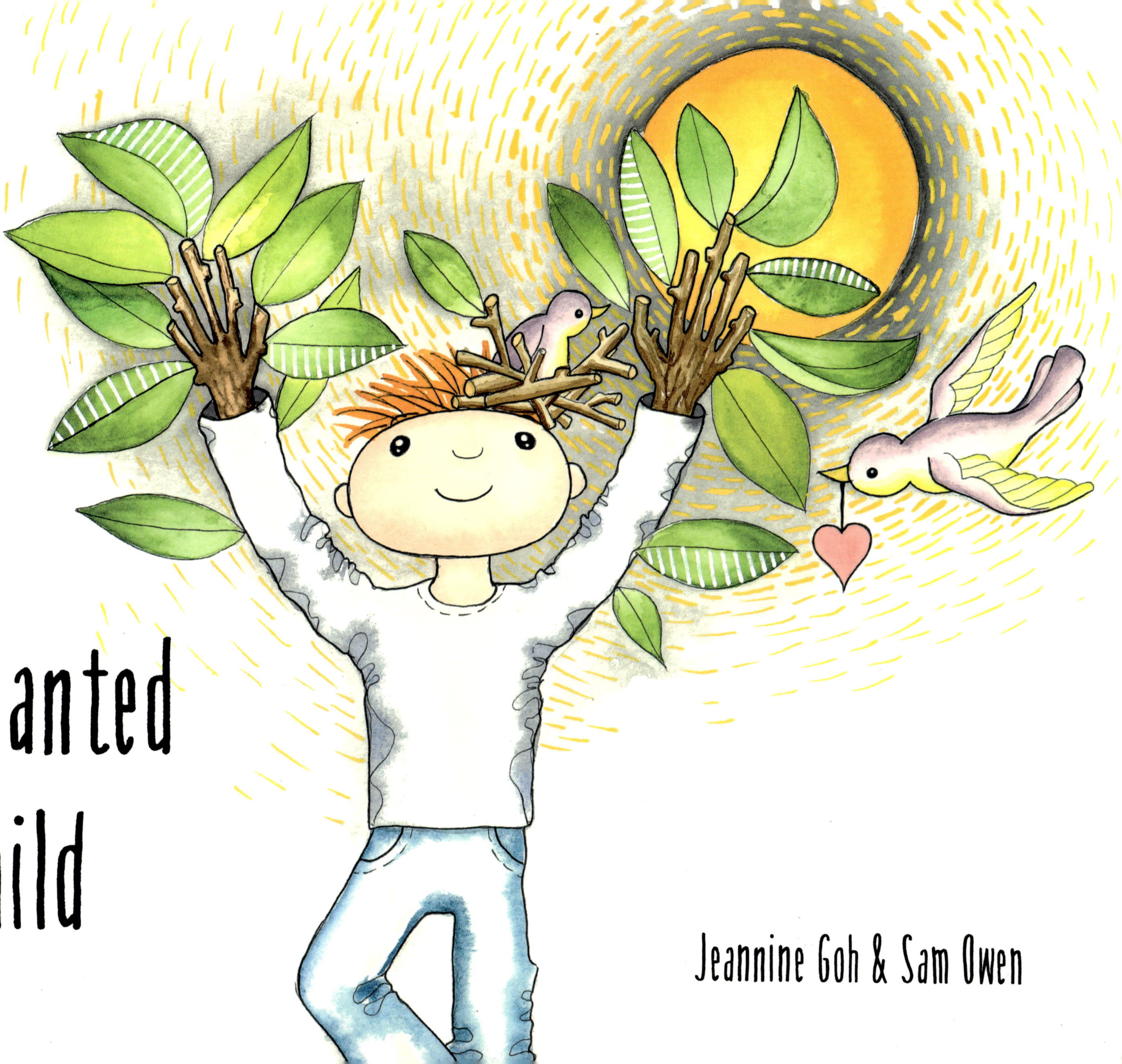

Jeannine Goh & Sam Owen

The Enchanted Child

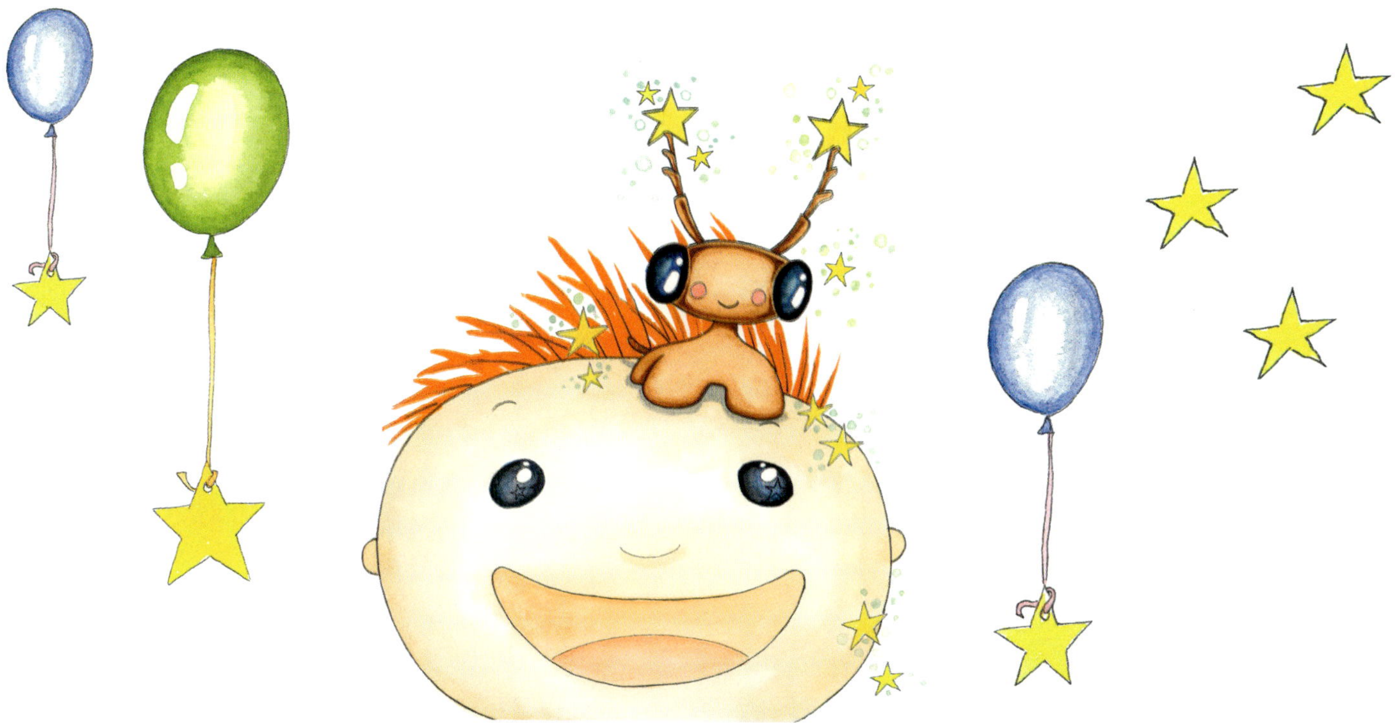

Written by Jeannine Goh
Illustrated by Sam Owen

AWESPACE

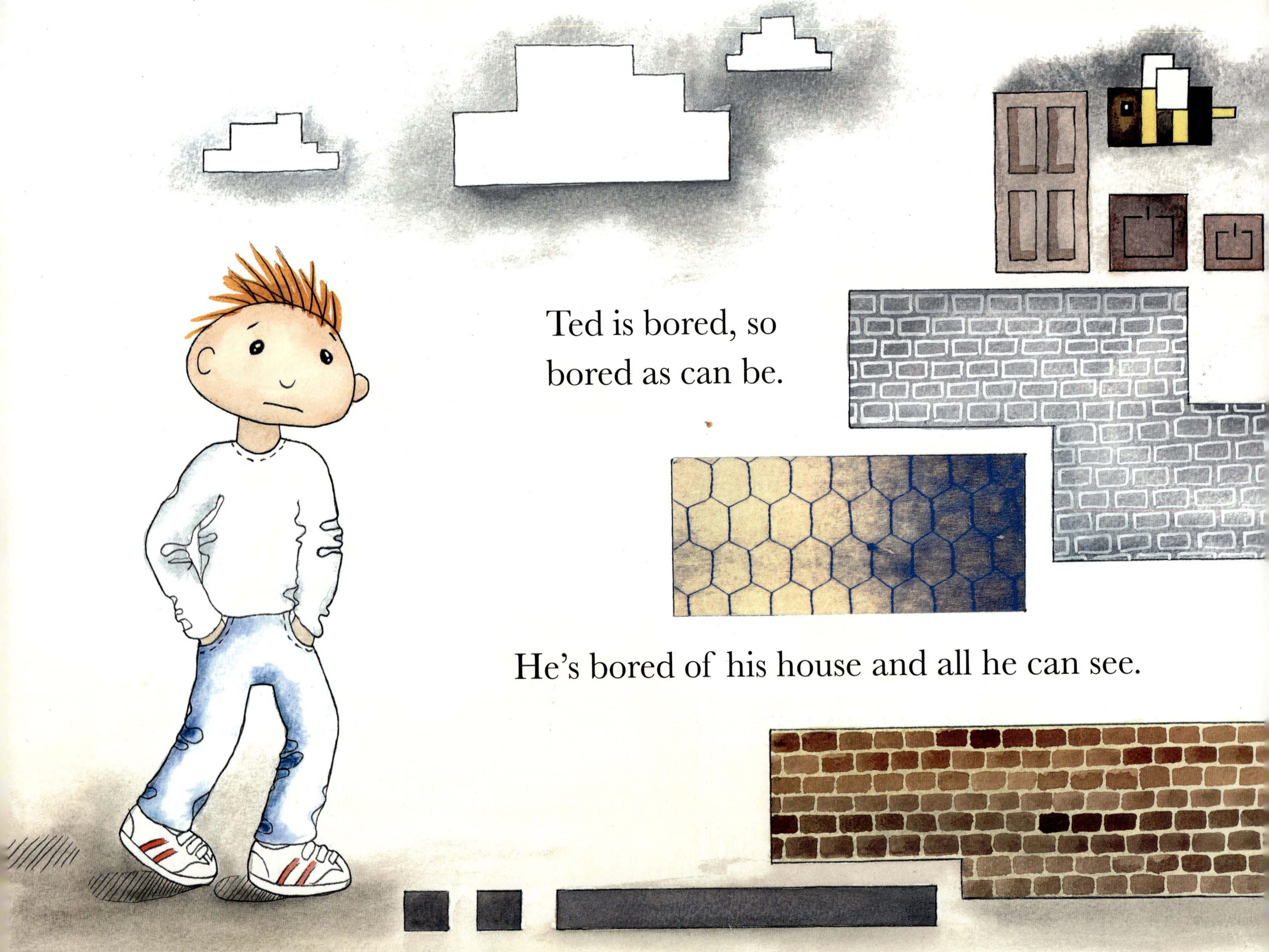

Ted is bored, so
bored as can be.

He's bored of his house and all he can see.

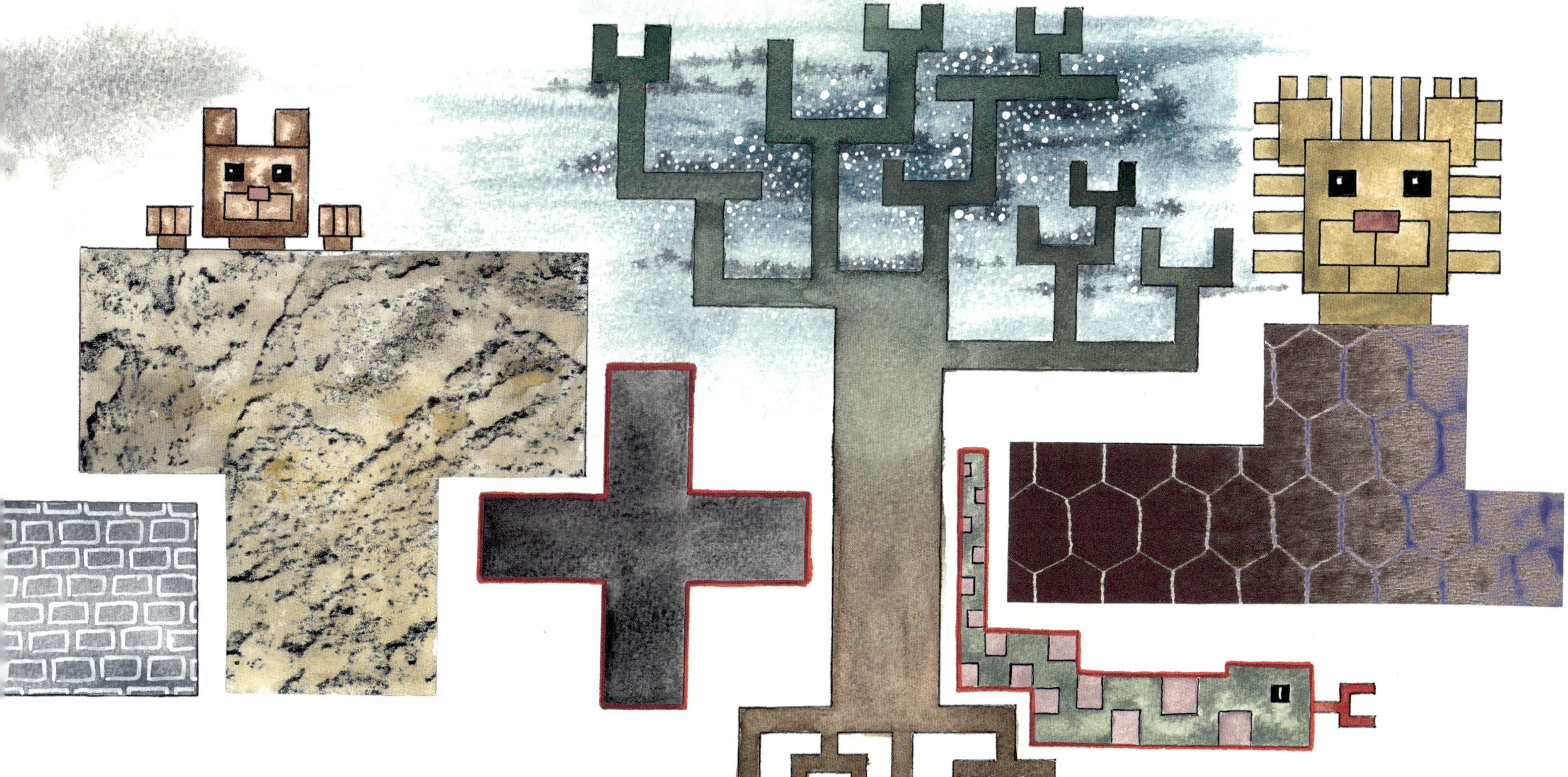

He's bored of his feet,

bored of his nose,

bored of his tongue

and bored of his toes.

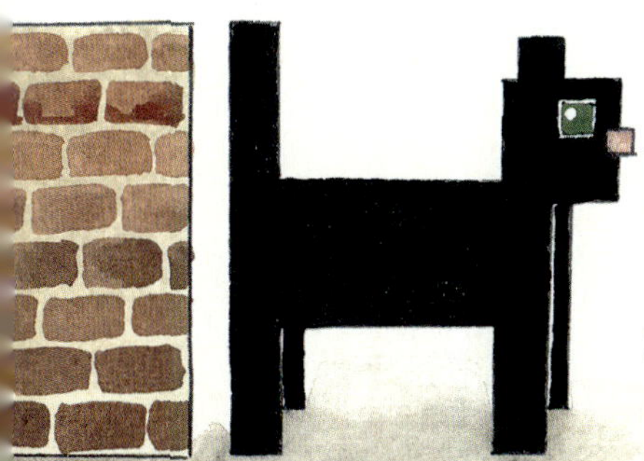

He… is…

bored of being

bored!

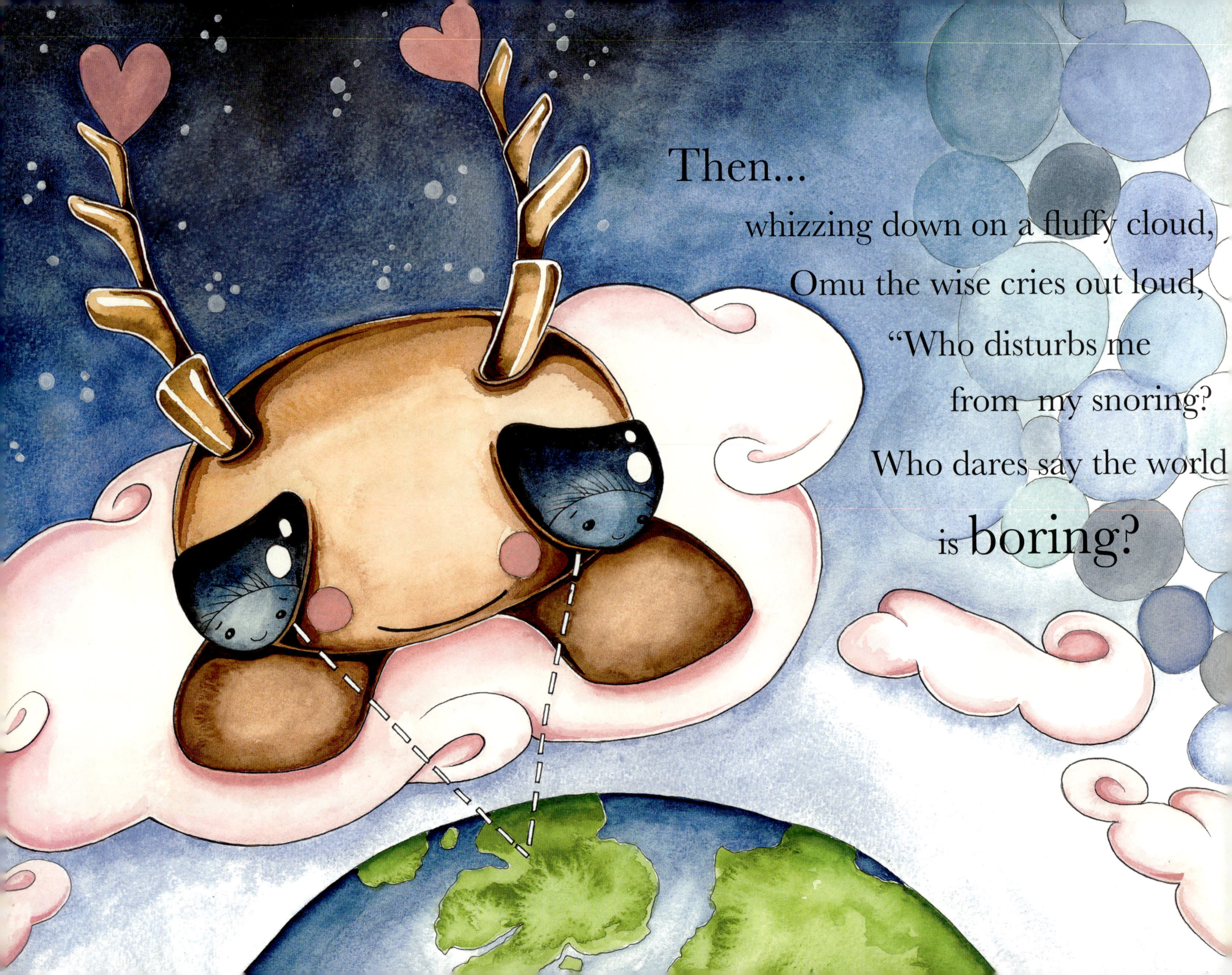

Then...

whizzing down on a fluffy cloud,

Omu the wise cries out loud,

“Who disturbs me

from my snoring?

Who dares say the world

is **boring?**

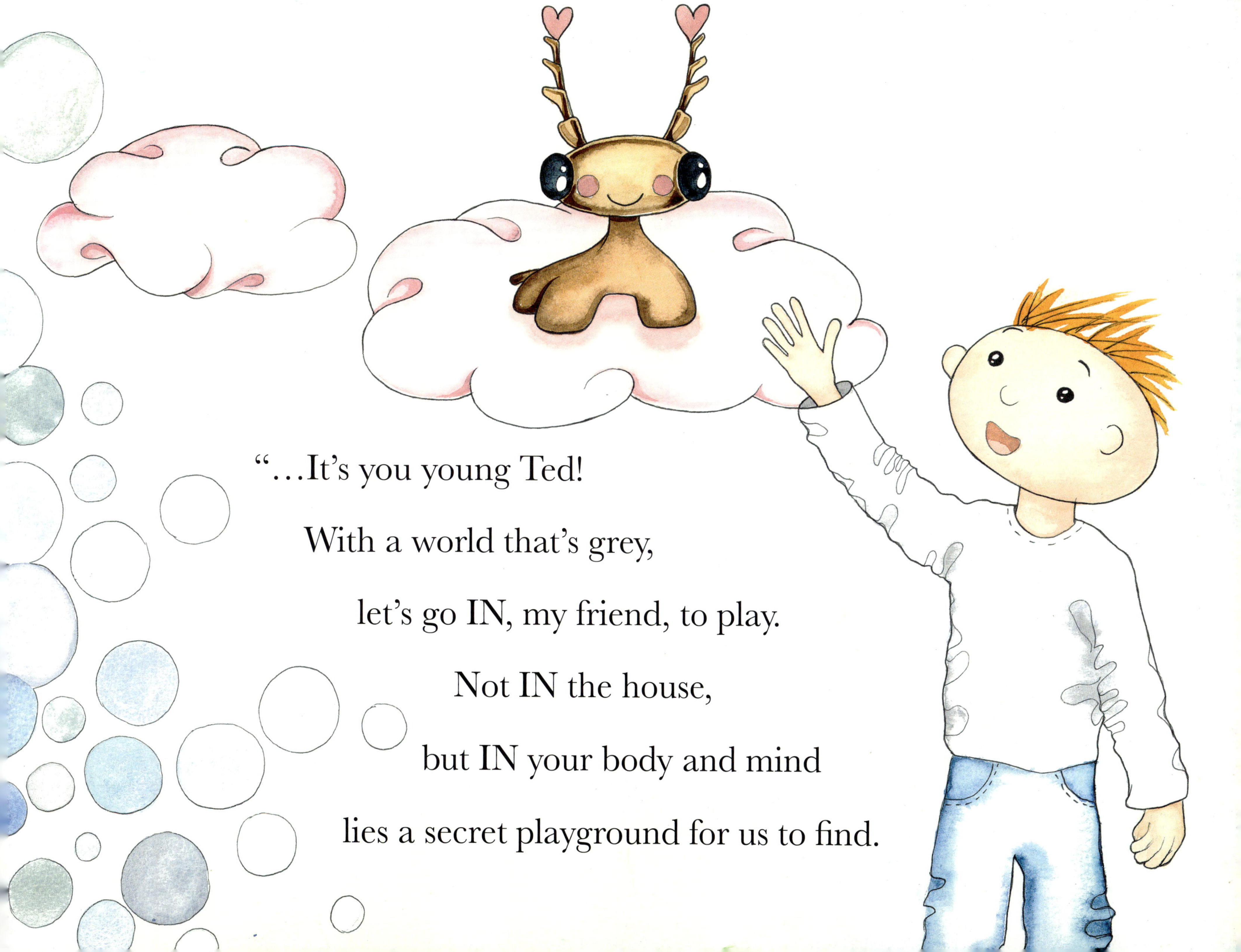

"…It's you young Ted!

With a world that's grey,

let's go IN, my friend, to play.

Not IN the house,

but IN your body and mind

lies a secret playground for us to find.

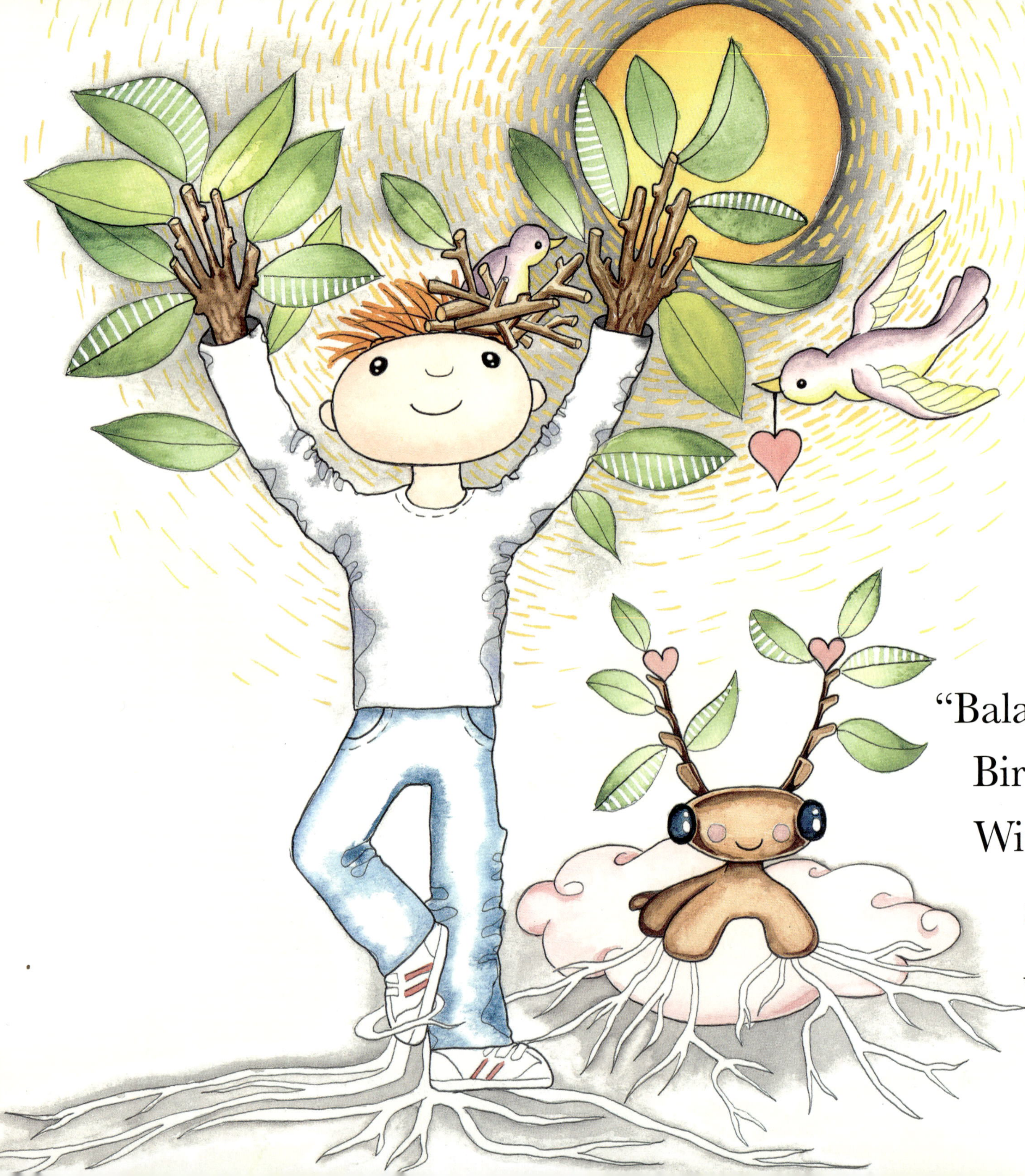

"Come…
Root your feet
within the ground.
Grow tall with me,
look all around.
You are powerful,
super-strong,
your body is in tune
with nature's song.

"Balance with me; be a tree.
Birds flutter our melody.
With a beat of the heart
and a magic blow,
we're animals now…
stars of a show!

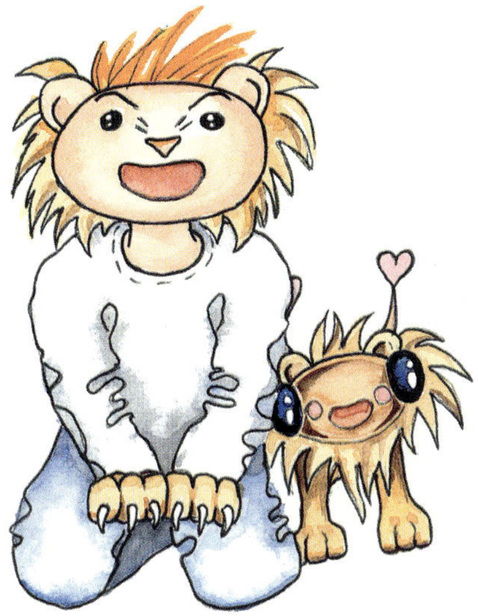

“I lead!

I’m a lion and I ROAR with pride…

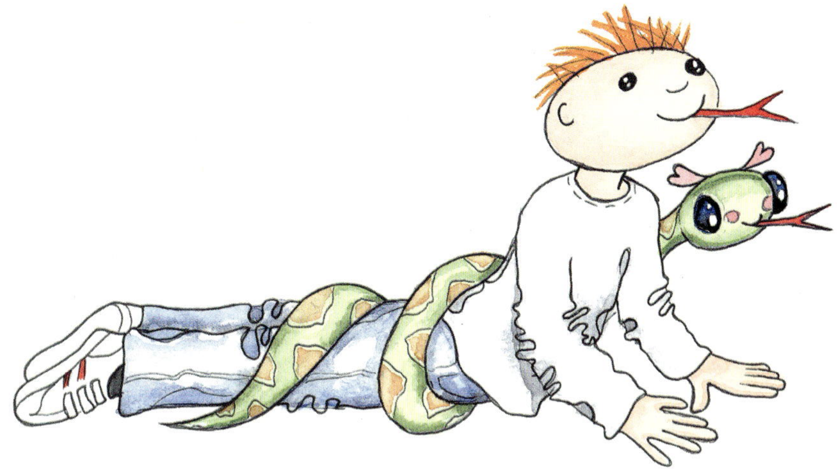

Mysterious cobra

with a HISS from the side.

Dog adds the backing

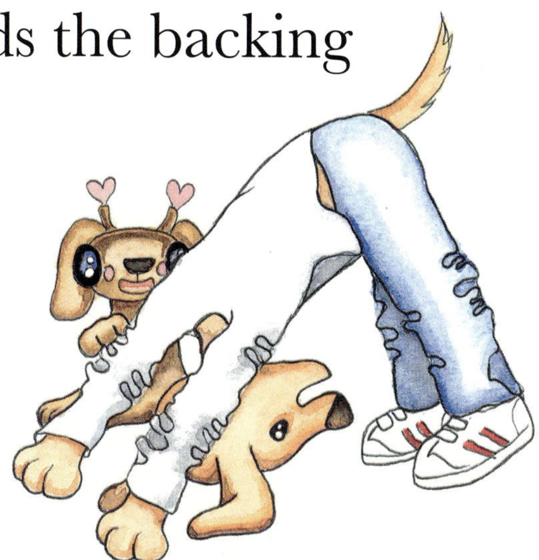

with a gruffly YAP!

Cat’s rhythmic slink

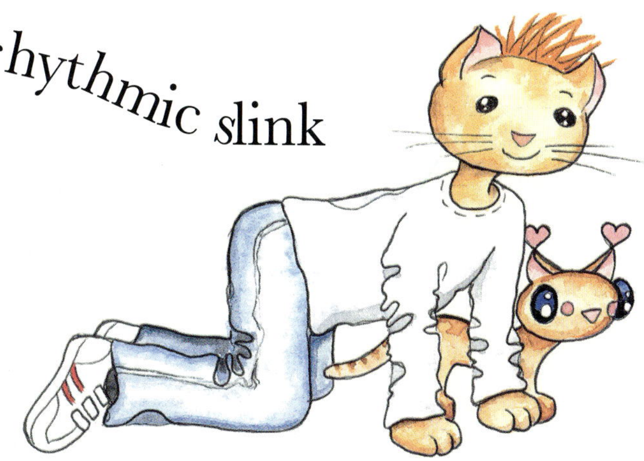

beats out a RAP!

"Buzzy Bee buzzes,

follow me

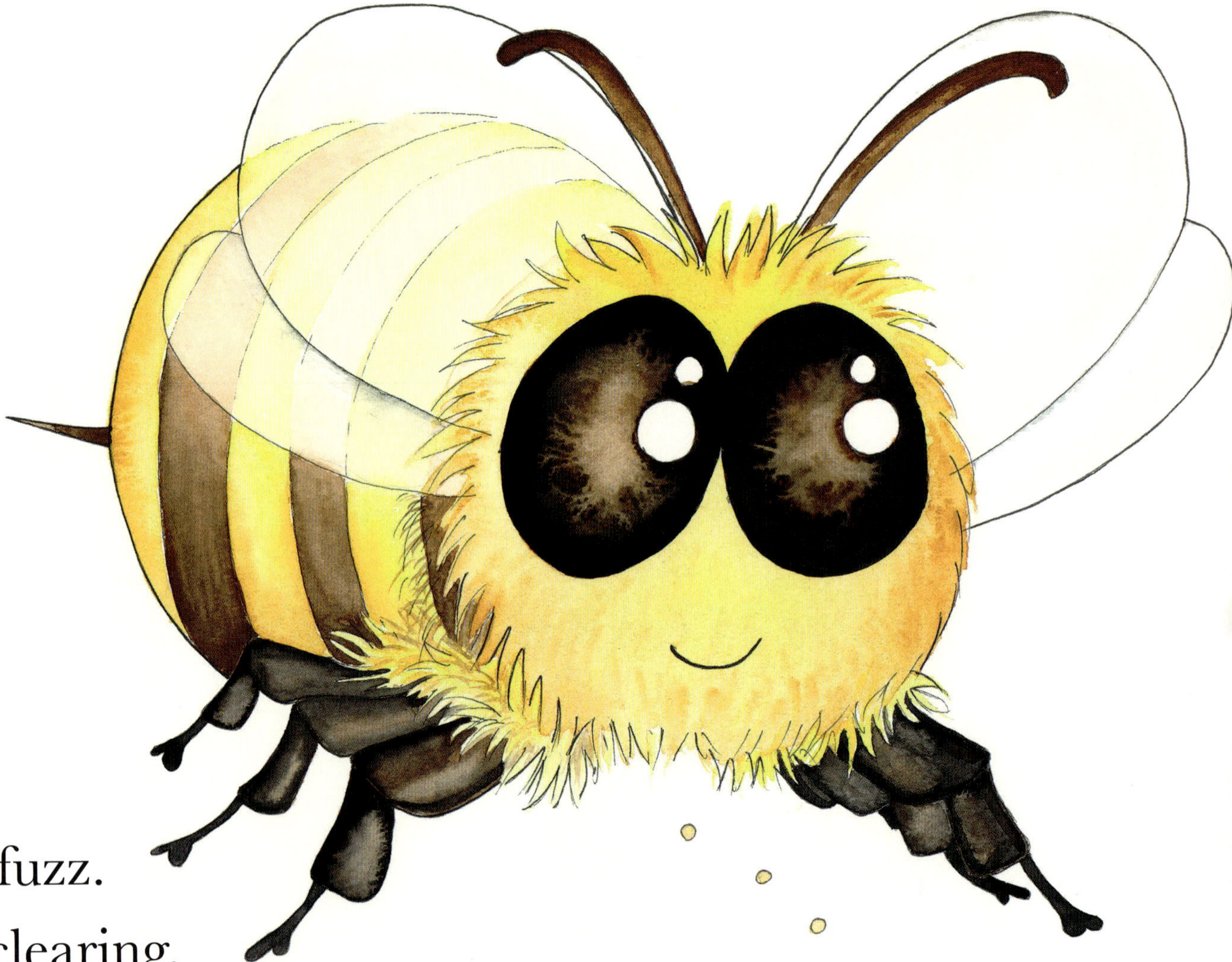

Buzz along, come be a bee.
Softly hum a gentle buzz,
it stills the wild mind's fuzzy fuzz.
Ears prick up, your mind is clearing,
activate...
SUPER-SONIC HEARING!

"Now, one more skill.

Stretch fingers out in front of your eyes.

Keep focus in front,

but take hands to the side.

If you can see hands

left and right.

Yes! You've done it!

SUPER-BRIGHT SIGHT!"

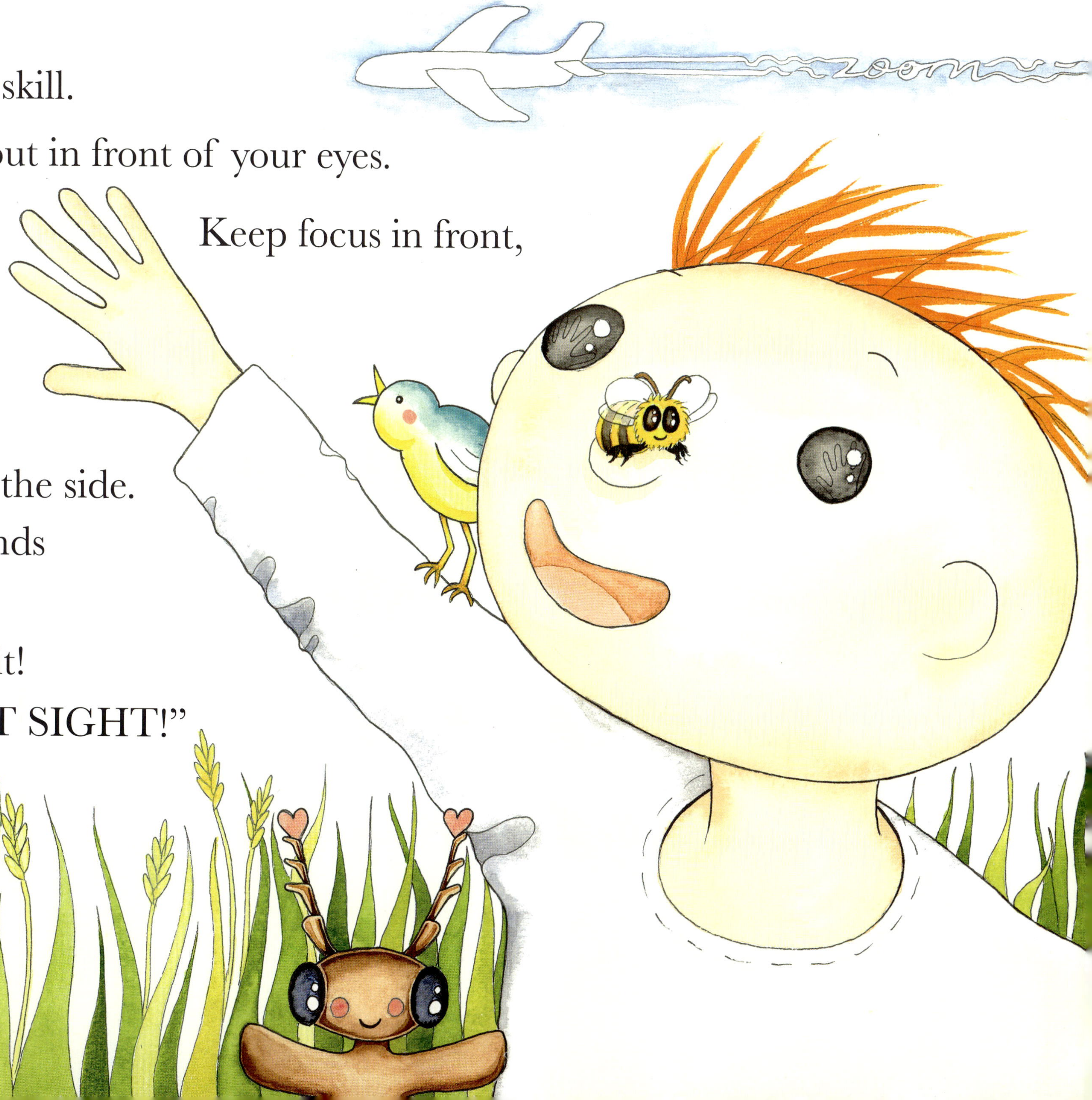

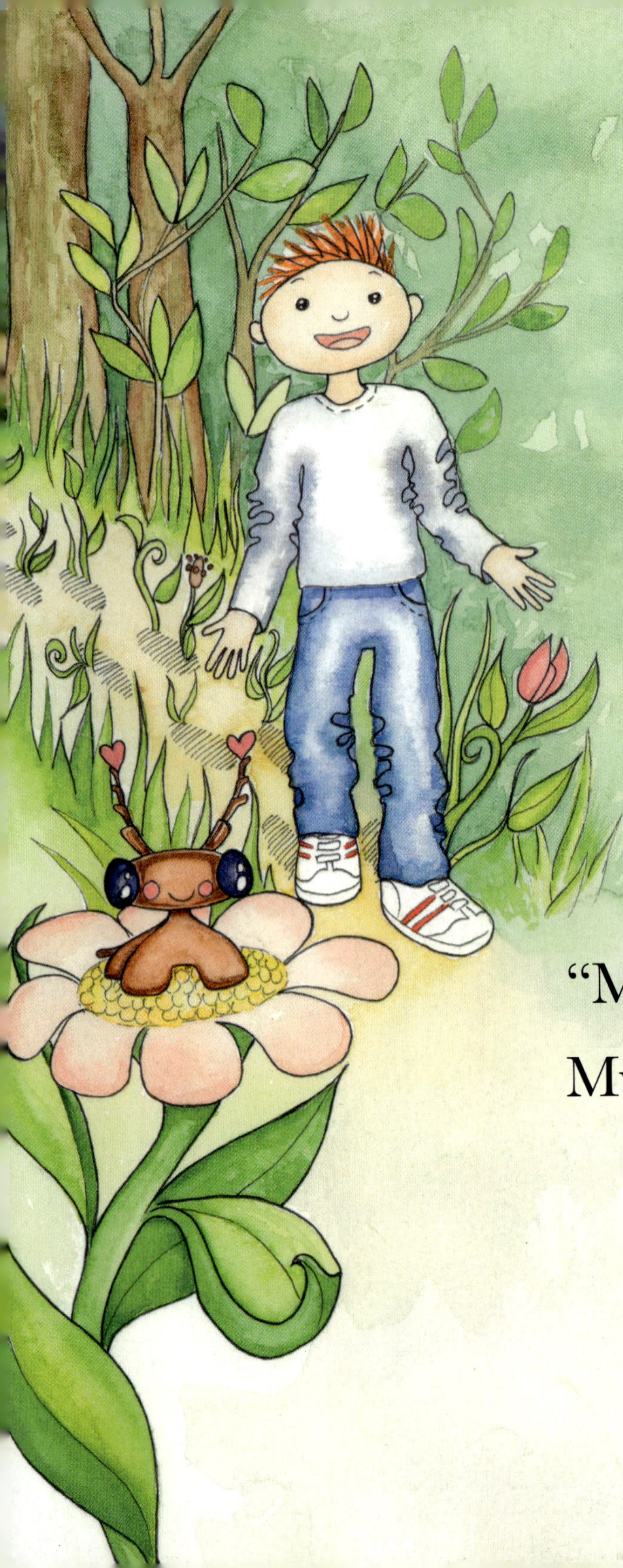

Then...
Ted spots over there,
with his super-bright eyes,
a beautiful girl.
Giant tears she cries.

"My name is Sal and I'm terribly sad.
My birthday's forgotten
and I feel so bad."

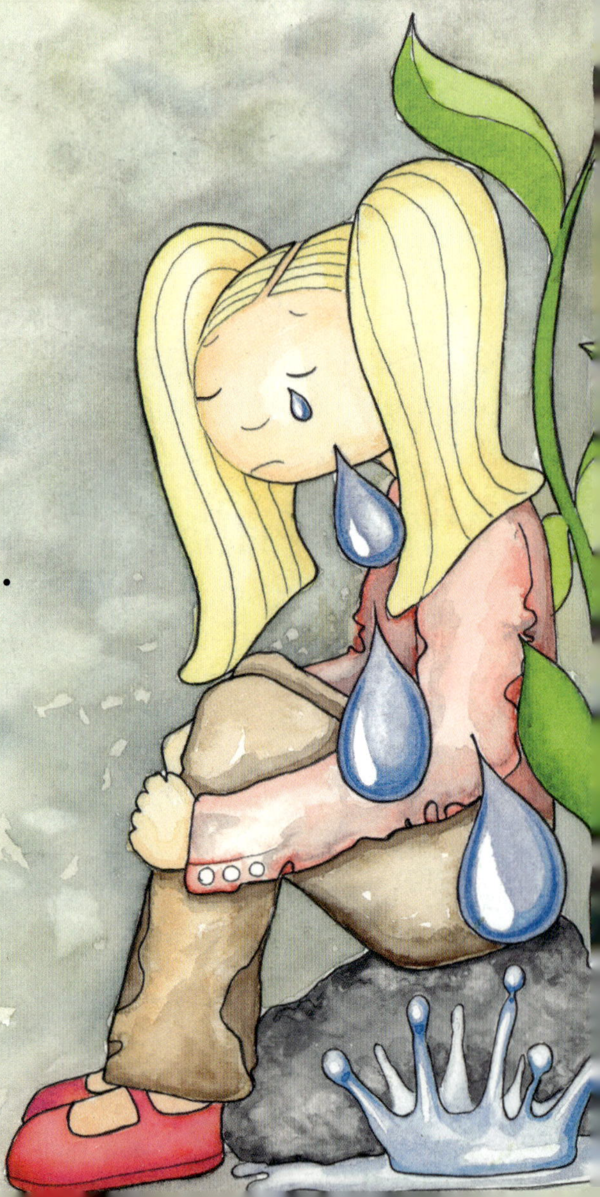

“Please my beauty cry no more,
it hurts me to see your red eyes
and cheeks all sore.
I’ve learnt these skills
and have new inner power.
I can share and teach you
in less than an hour.
Then together I promise you
...that’s if we believe...
The best birthday party
a girl could ever receive.”

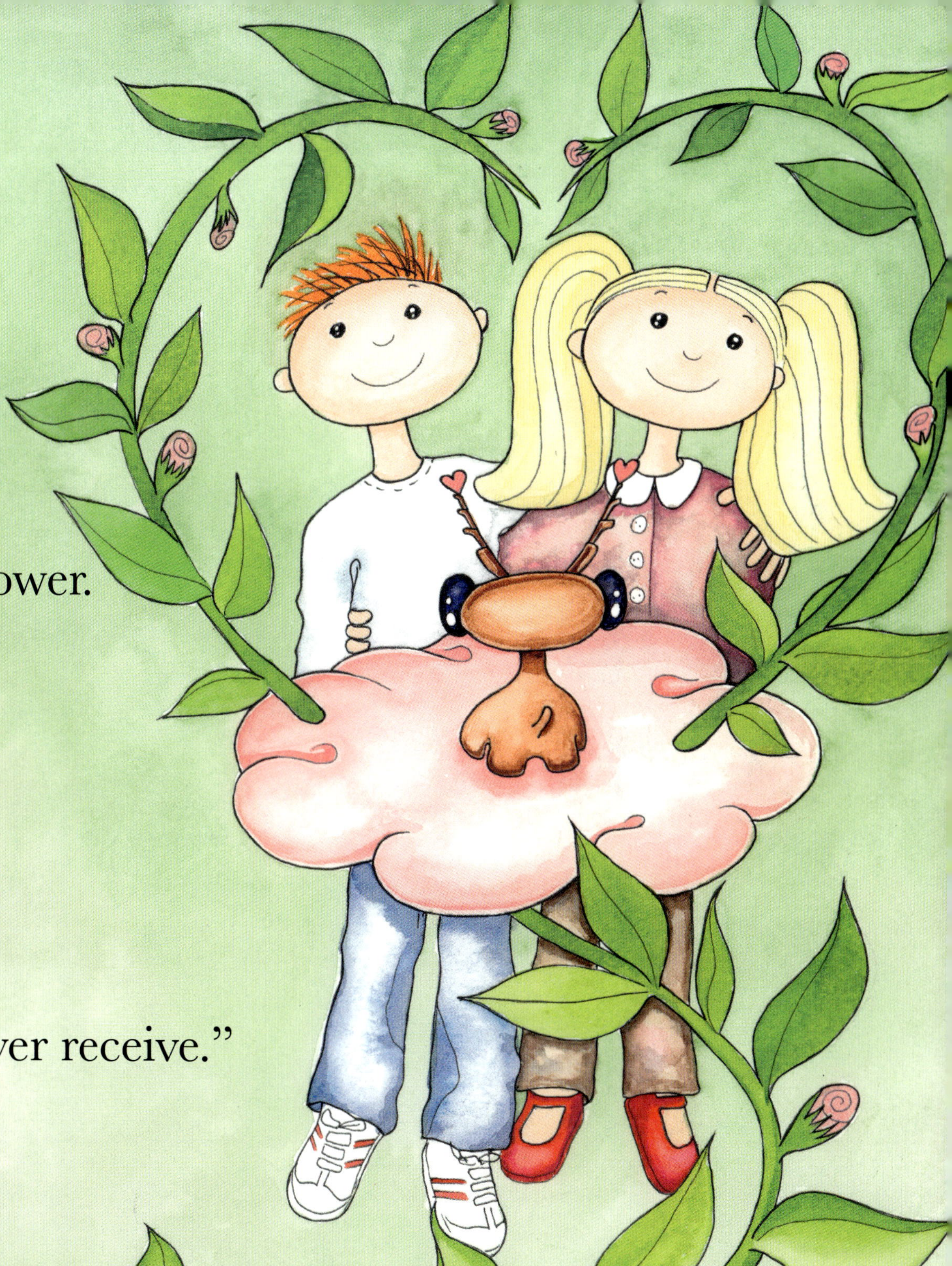

Ted scratches his head and tries to recall
Omu's super powers, to teach Sal them all.
Can you be brilliant, and help if you will?
Try to remember each super skill.

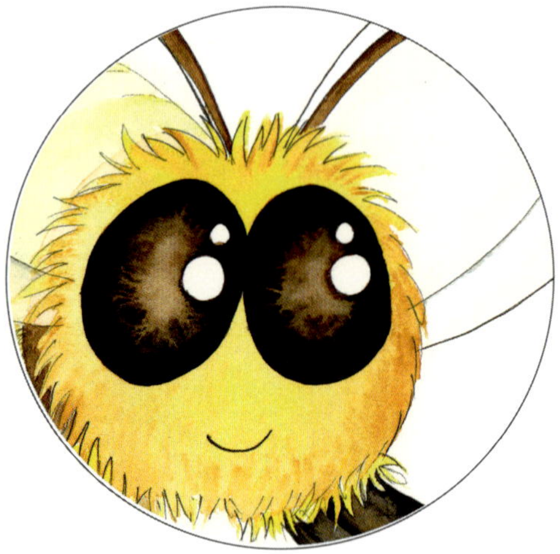

SUPER-SONIC HEARING
detects anything nearing.

Be an instinctive knight
with SUPER-BRIGHT SIGHT.

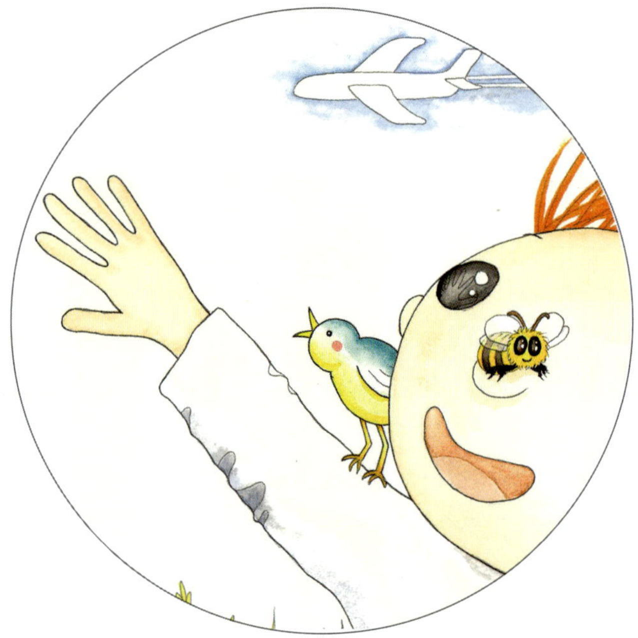

Power up to be SUPER-flexi and STRONG.
You'll feel so amazing and it doesn't take long!

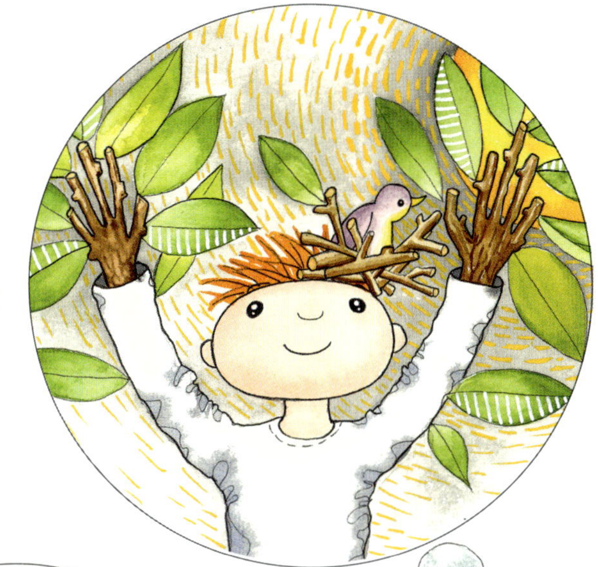

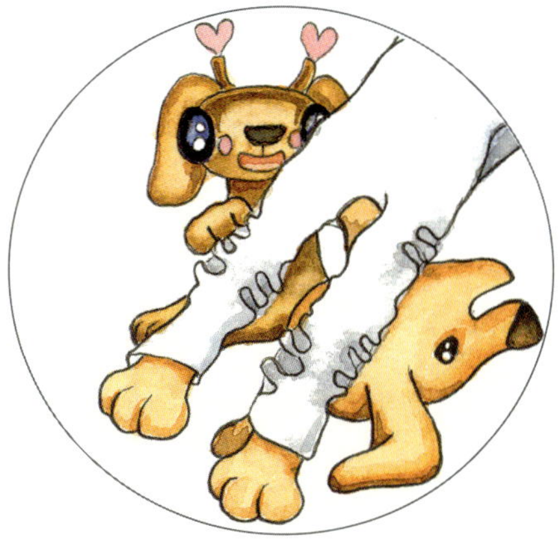

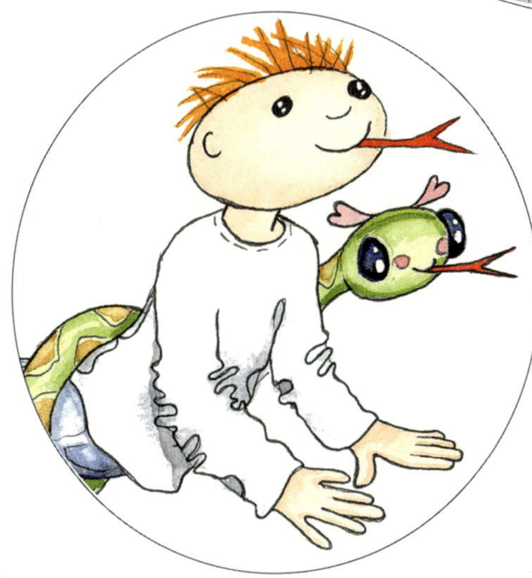

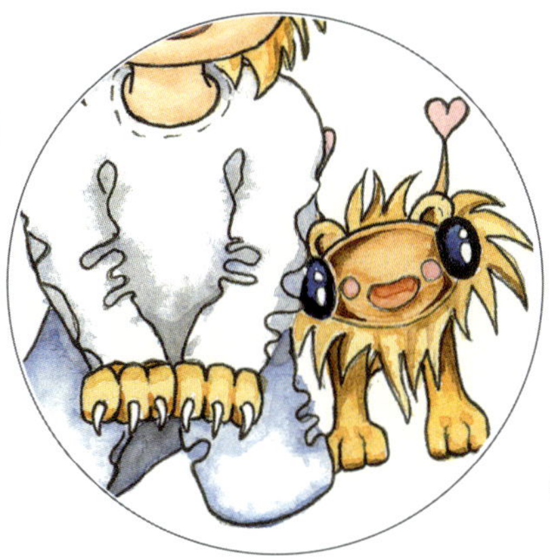

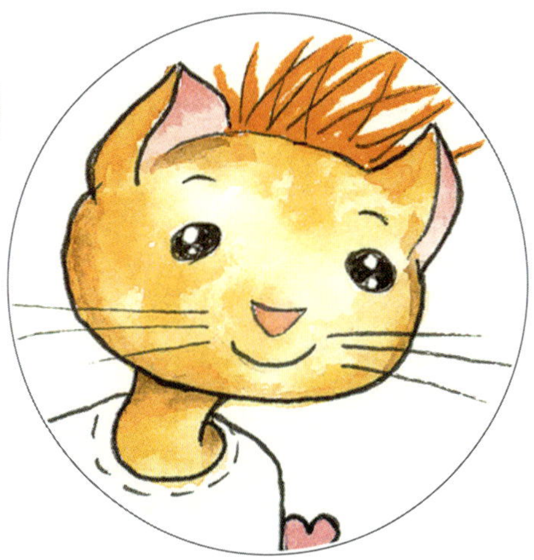

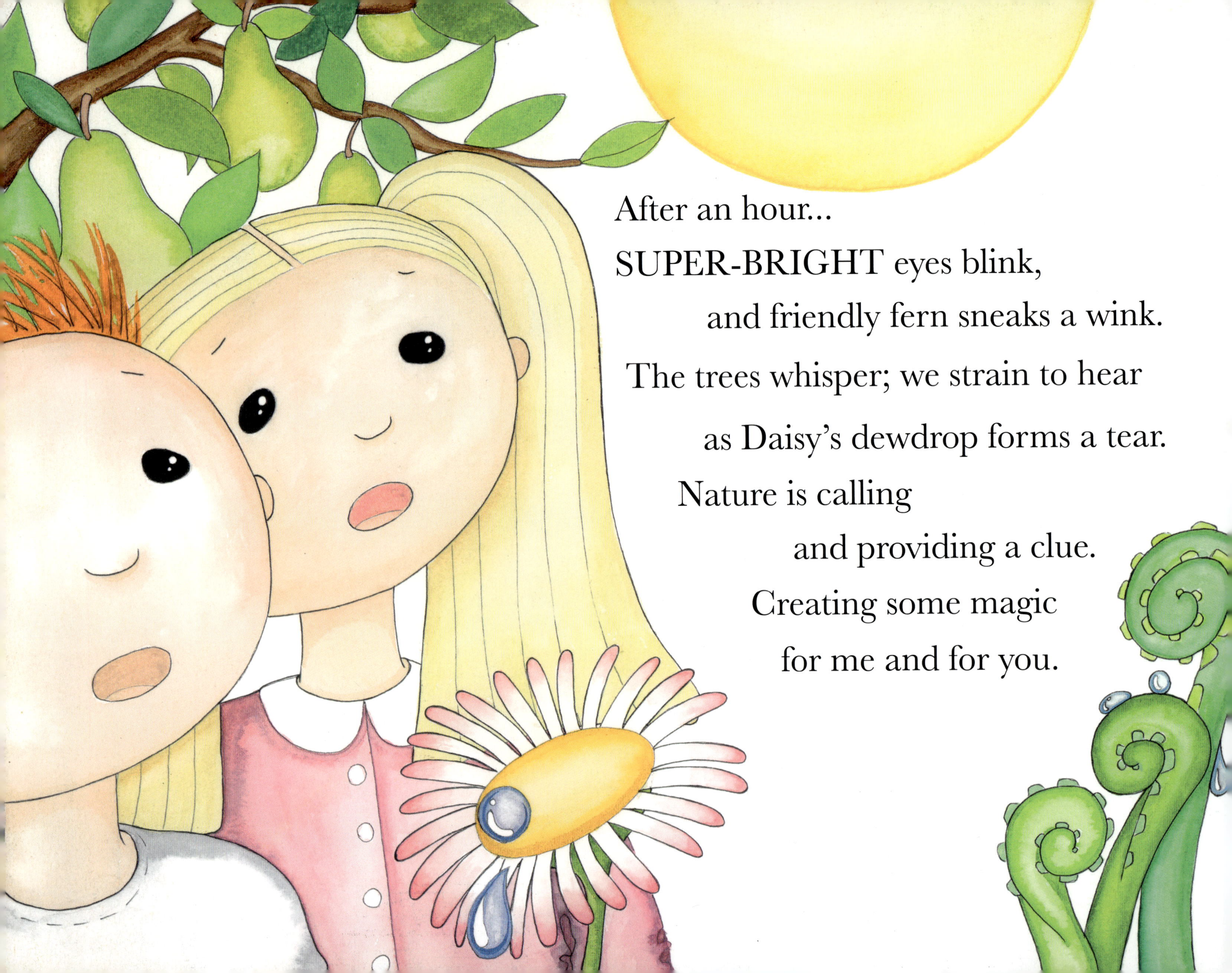

After an hour...
SUPER-BRIGHT eyes blink,
and friendly fern sneaks a wink.
The trees whisper; we strain to hear
as Daisy's dewdrop forms a tear.
Nature is calling
and providing a clue.
Creating some magic
for me and for you.

Then…
Hidden from sight
and overgrown,
a lonely apple tree
lets out a groan.

"Delicious apples each year I bear.
They all go rotten before I can share."

"Don't worry tree, we'll set you free,"
says Ted,
as the excited apples dance
around his head.

The branches bend...
the apples glint with glee.

"Happy birthday Sal…a gift…
YIPPEE!

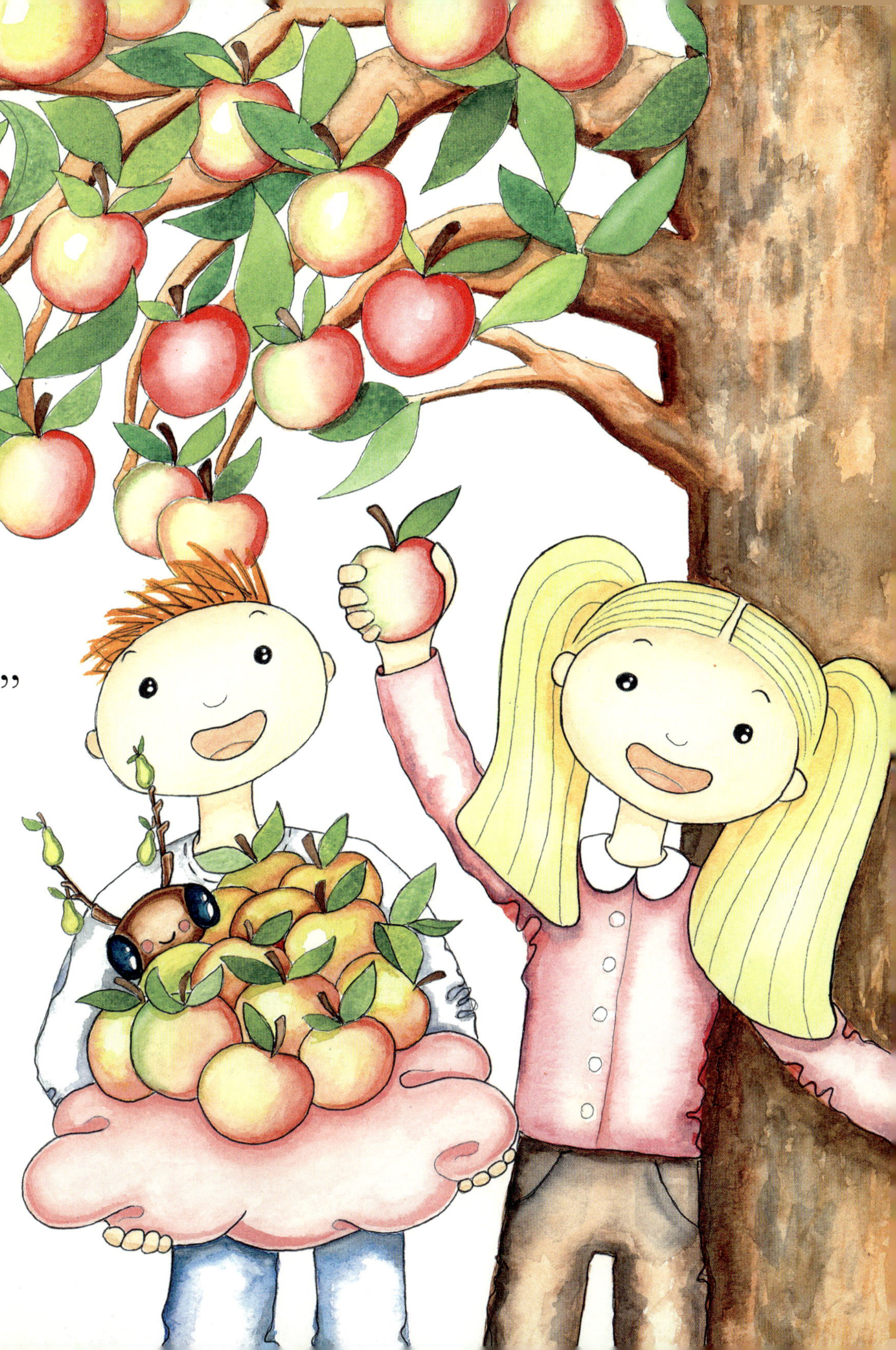

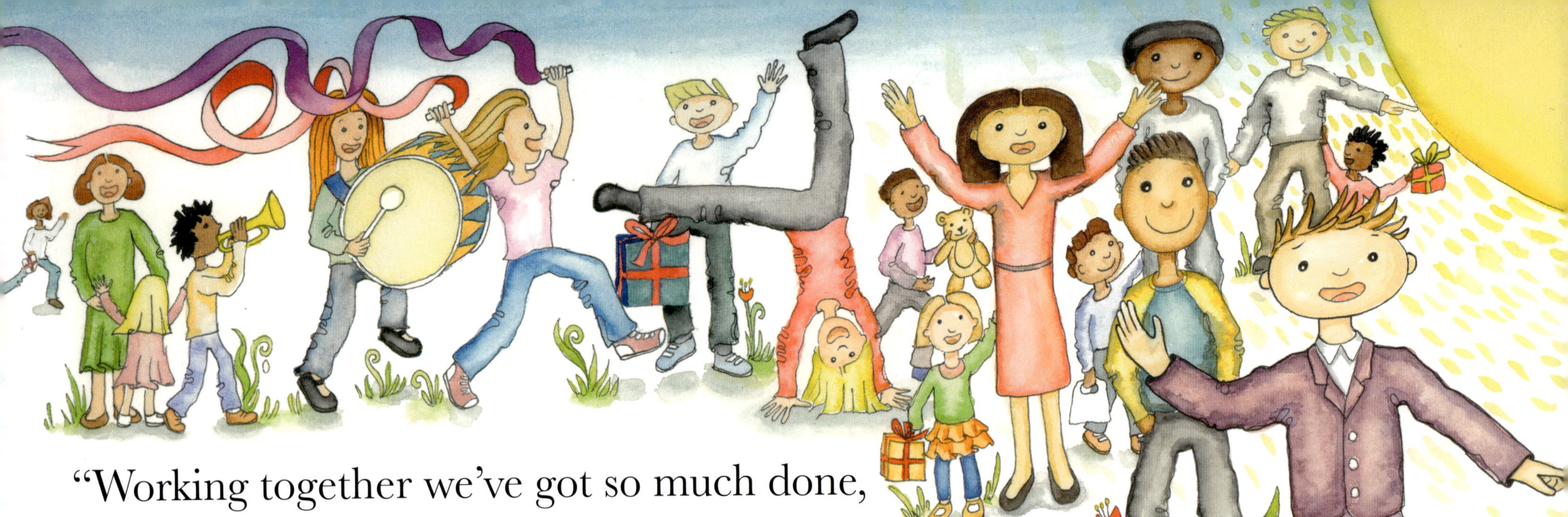

"Working together we've got so much done,
I feel so excited and out comes the sun!
Everything is unfolding just as it should.
A party is starting, I said that it would!
I feel it's as if, our world is aglow.
I can hear birthday music, come on let's go!"

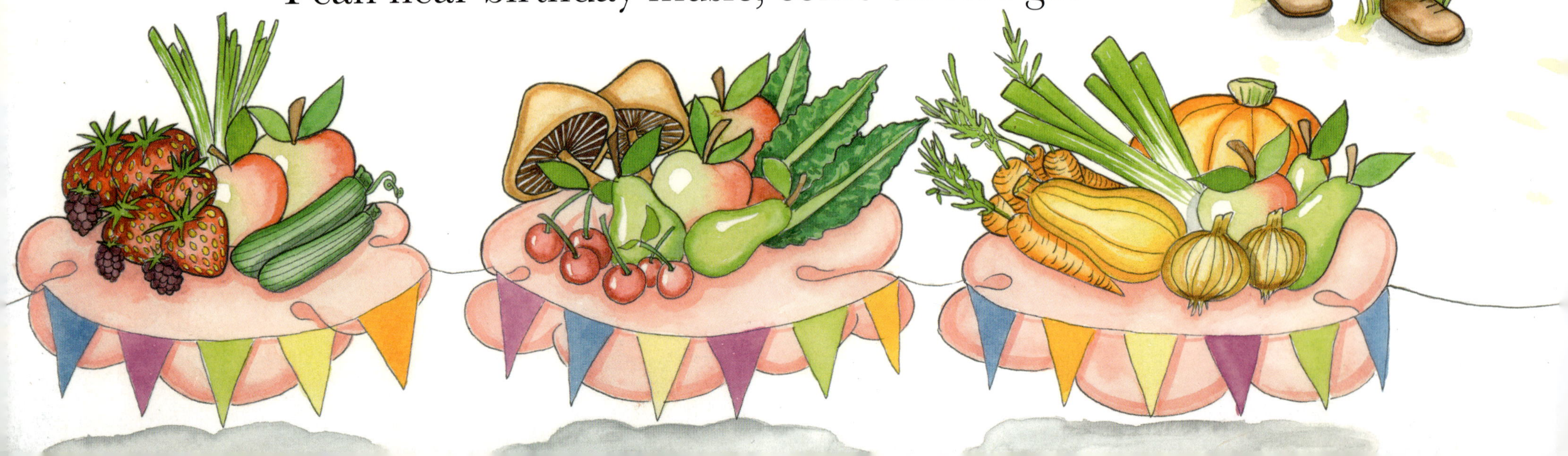

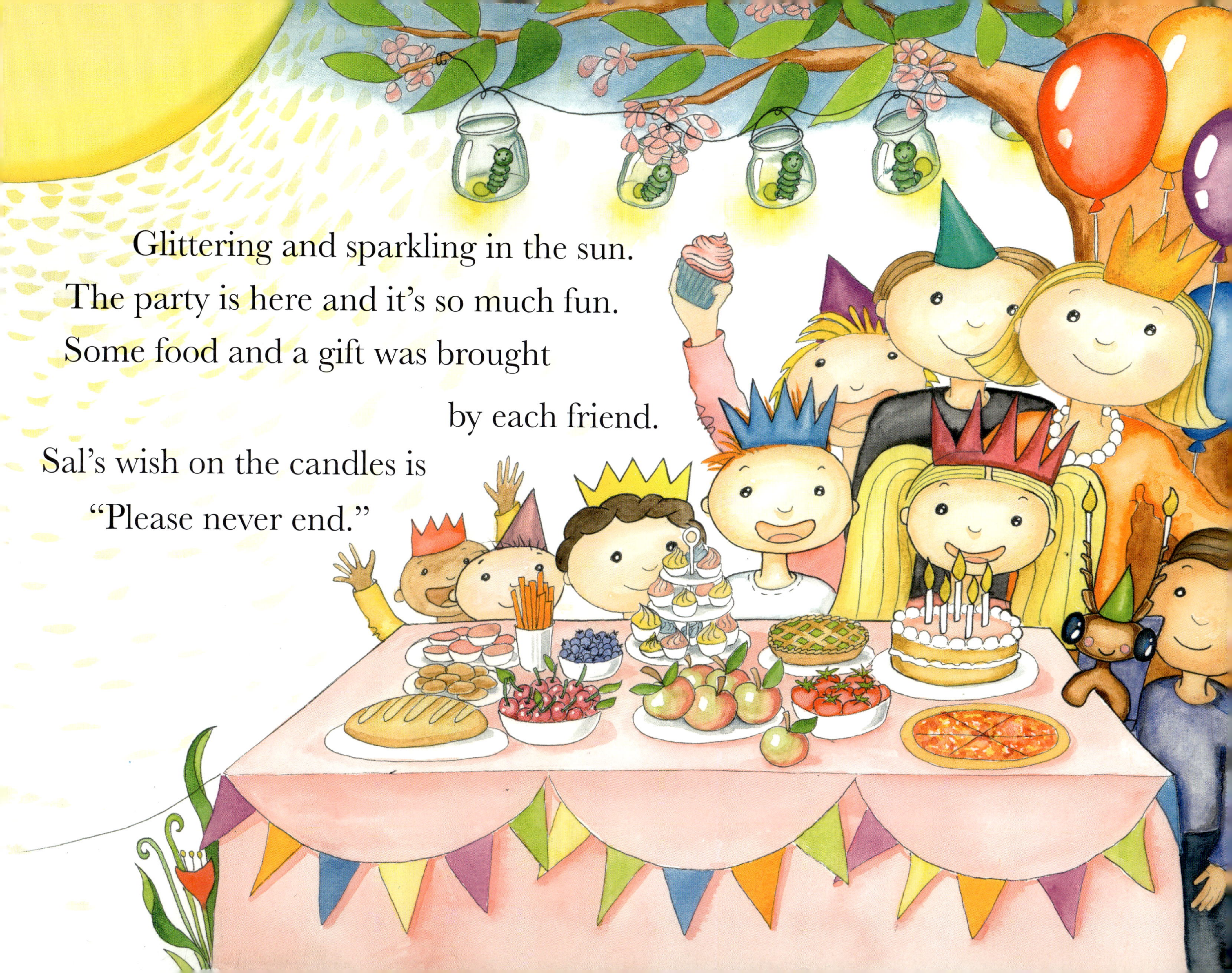

Glittering and sparkling in the sun.
The party is here and it's so much fun.
Some food and a gift was brought
by each friend.
Sal's wish on the candles is
"Please never end."

Dancing and singing and chatting to all,
my goodness me…we're having a ball!
Everyone has come from every land.
Everyone is friends and holding my hand.
Celebrating life, a birthday…the earth,
this journey has brought me such self-worth.

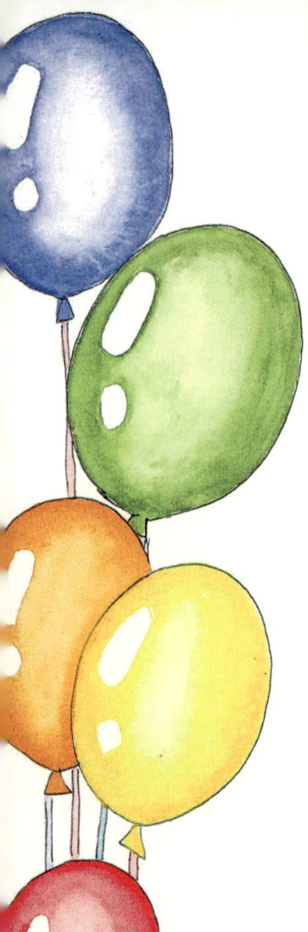
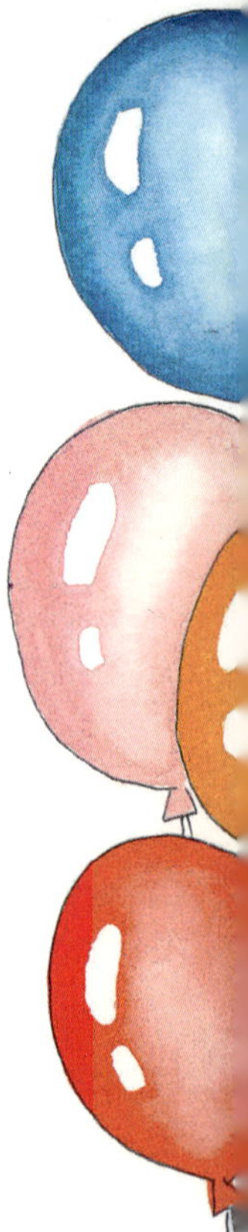
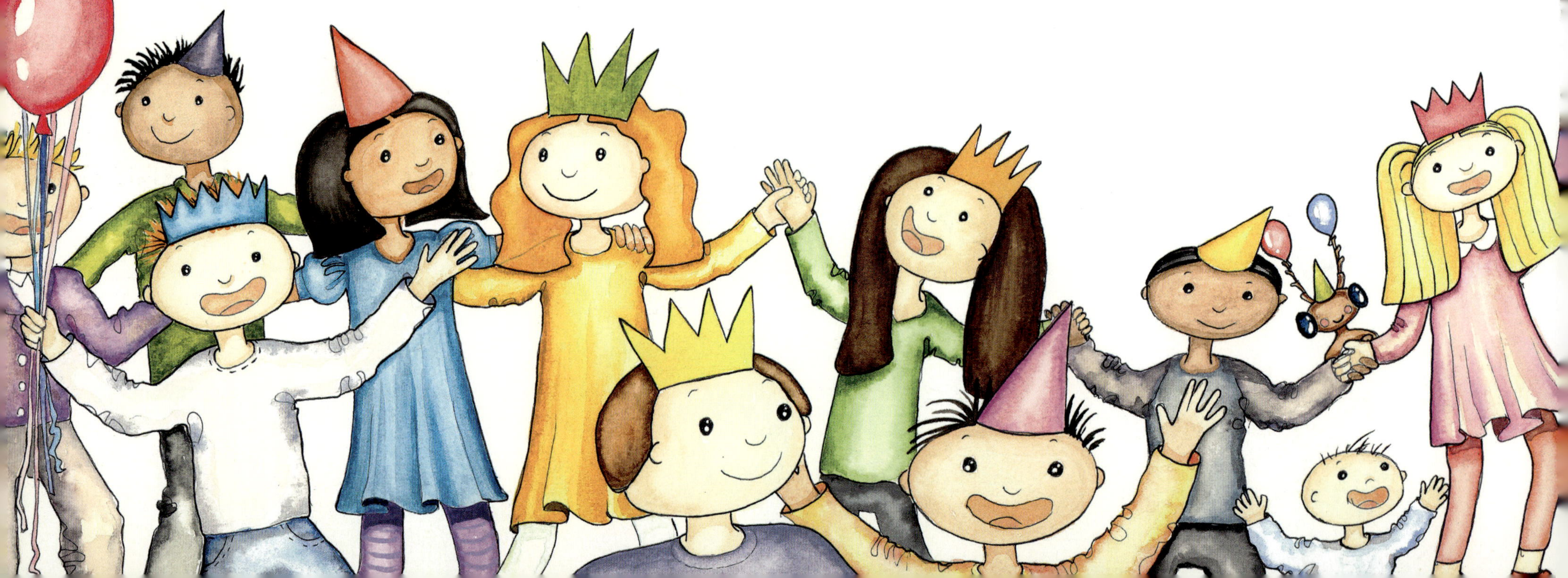

“Thank you...thank YOU,

may I never forget…

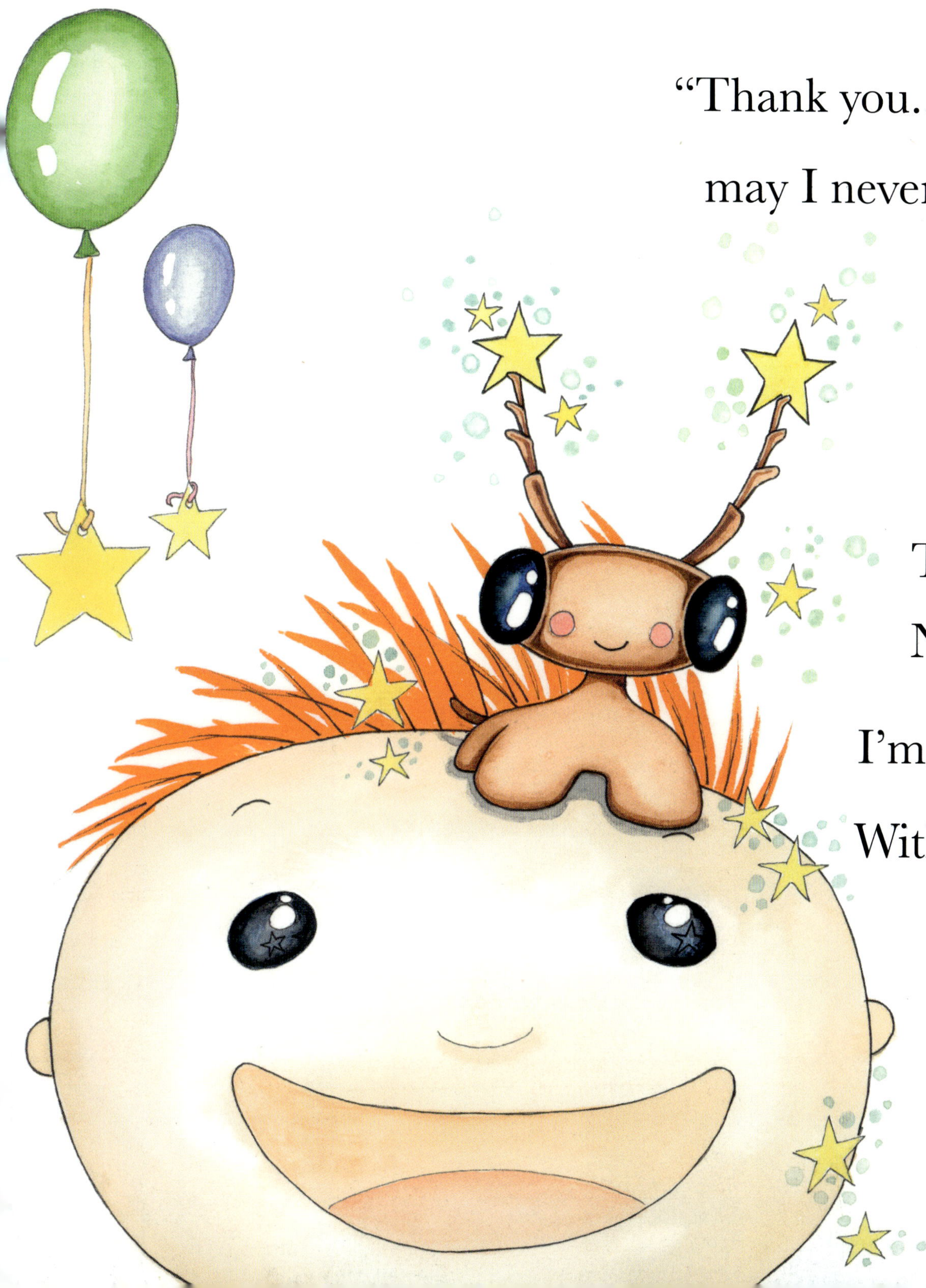

“With these powers I can see.

I have become a MAGIC ME.

There is no wand, there is no trick.

No pazazz or magician’s stick.

I’m here I’m living in a beautiful land,

With opportunity and hope all around.

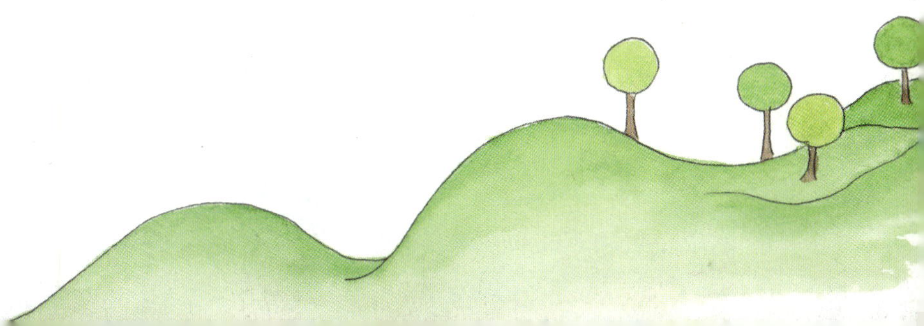

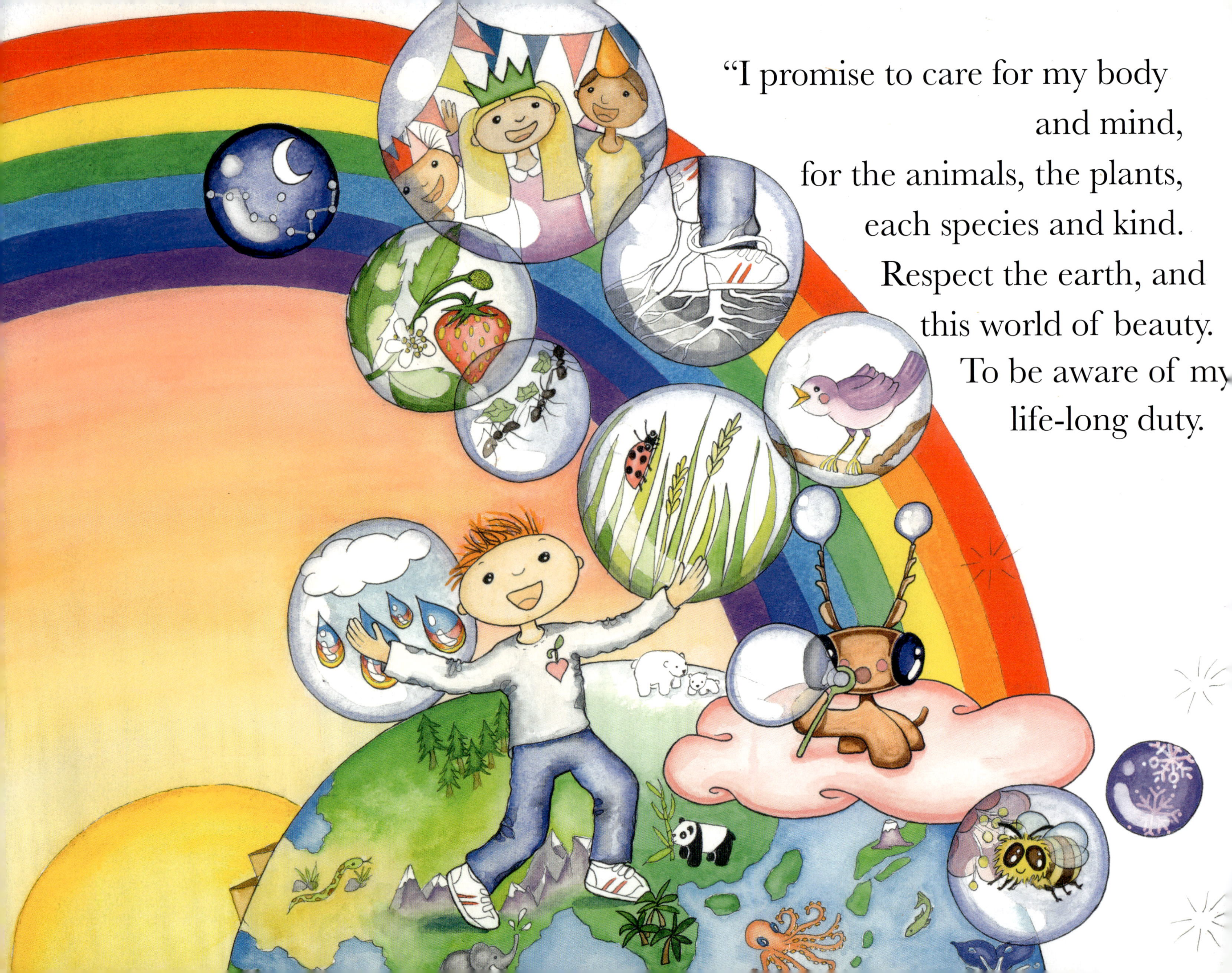

"I promise to care for my body
and mind,
for the animals, the plants,
each species and kind.
Respect the earth, and
this world of beauty.
To be aware of my
life-long duty.

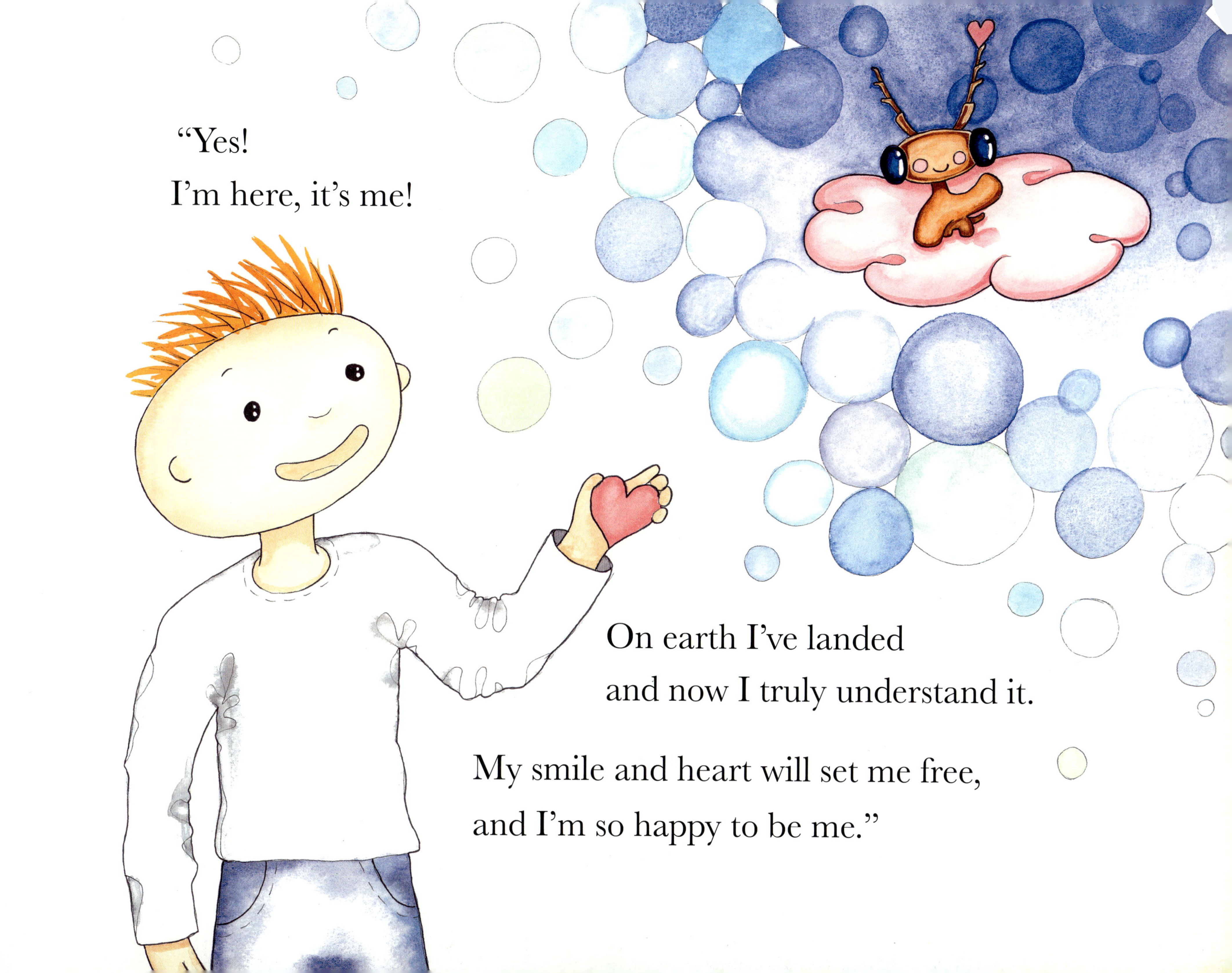

"Yes!
I'm here, it's me!

On earth I've landed
and now I truly understand it.

My smile and heart will set me free,
and I'm so happy to be me."

Enchanting our children

Raising children is notoriously difficult. As well as the sleepless nights, the constant tidying and washing, and supporting our children through their more challenging behavioural phases, we are also living through a huge technological revolution. Our children are therefore bombarded by messages from the television and the Internet, and we as parents receive constant conflicting messages about parenting.

We live in a consumerist society where our children are persuaded to want more and more, and we live more isolated and housebound lives, with weak community ties. I'm afraid to say that modern-day culture inspires and excites our children with many misleading messages, which do not promote their well-being. The latest child well-being statistics and research make sombre reading and I believe that our children need our help.

I truly feel that our children deserve a kinder approach to their development, and that we must carefully consider how we introduce them to the world. We need to gather together to ensure that the messages we convey to our children are empowering, life-affirming, consistent and based on sensible morals and values. We, as parents, adults and educators, need to take back the ownership of deciding what is best for our children.

In front of us lies a great opportunity for change; a chance to ensure that our young children, who come into this world full of excitement and wonder, stay enchanted rather than become disenchanted. As a parent, psychologist, practical philosopher, yoga teacher and workshop leader for children and parents, I draw together over twenty years of thinking, researching and practice to share a vision of how we can come together to cultivate, nurture and raise enchanted children.

What is an enchanted child?

An enchanted child is delighted by the world around them. They notice, appreciate and are connected to all aspects of life. They are amazed by their bodies which they treat with respect. They are enraptured by the scope of their minds and all they can achieve. They live from their hearts, love to care and share, and recognise the importance of community and working for the greater good. They look at nature with wonder and acknowledge the interconnection of everything. Excited by their own, and others', potential they are in awe of life, the world and the universe.

The enchanted child story

I believe cultivating these aspects in our children should be a priority, but I worry that such teachings are displaced in our culture and education system in favour of academic achievement. I therefore started to think carefully about how we could introduce life-lessons to children in a colourful way. I am now on a mission to raise a generation of healthy, happy and enchanted children.

Storytelling is one technique which, in my experience, can be transformative and can act as a gentle and subtle way to explore life with children. With all this in mind, I developed the Enchanted Child story which whisks your child away on a wondrous journey of discovery.

The story is fast-paced and is designed as a spark for further discussion. Importantly, embedded within its pages are various skills and techniques, that draw together ancient wisdom with the latest research in modern-day psychology. The book is based around a series of life-lessons (connecting with the body and mind; others and community; nature; and the wider world and cosmos) that can be used as a basis for exploration with your child. With the help of the illustrations, and with the following extra information, I hope this book will be a rich source of inspiration for you and your child.

Some of the techniques and wisdom within the book are inspired by the ancient art of yoga. Yoga is often associated with people bending and contorting their bodies, but actually yoga simply means to connect. As well as yoga encouraging a strong, healthy and supple body, it also teaches us how to settle the mind. This allows for the creation of more mindful connections. Yoga is therefore not just a physical practice but one which encourages self-awareness and compassion to promote a strong, calm and flexible mind.

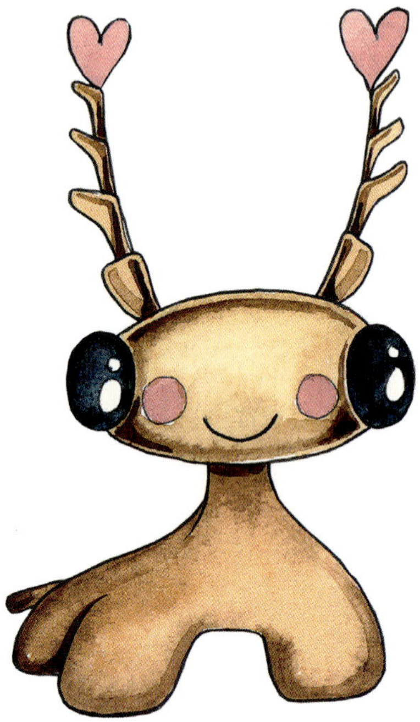

The guide in the book is called Omu, who teaches a range of skills and techniques. These techniques are fantastic for the body and mind, and also encourage deeper reflection. Significantly, the name Omu is derived from OM, which is an important word in yoga that represents the vibration of the universe. Saying, or chanting, OM helps with mental focus, while the resonating and vibrating effect further calms and settles the mind.

In the beginning of the story it is lovely to encourage the children to call Omu by singing 'auh-mm--moo, auh-mm-moo'. It is very relaxing to sing or chant this, and you can experiment with different tones (how low or high can you chant Omu?) and intonations. Singing also actively engages your child in the story.

Looking after the mind and body

The book introduces your child to six simple yoga postures that each have notable physical, mental and emotional benefits. These are known as mountain, tree, lion, cobra, dog, and cat pose.

I find it useful to ask children to grow into the postures and I encourage them to move in slow motion. This helps maximise their control over their bodies. You can also ask them to grow into a pose with an inhalation, and then relax and rest in the pose as they exhale. I will try to give detailed instructions to enable you and your child to fully explore these postures and breathing.

Mountain pose

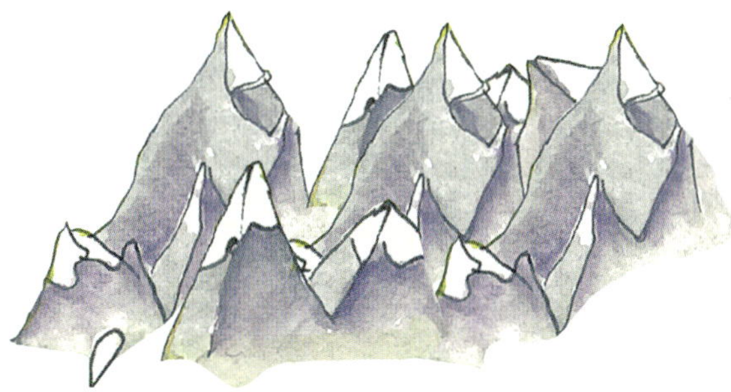

To begin, encourage your child to wiggle their feet and toes (socks off), and try to feel their feet on the ground. Encourage them to imagine they have deep roots which grow down from their feet into the ground to create a strong and firm base.

Ask them to imagine that their lungs are a balloon and as they breathe in, the balloon expands and they grow taller. As the crown reaches up towards the sky, ask them to simultaneously grow their roots longer and deeper into the earth. This lengthens the spine allowing your child to grow taller and taller. As they exhale, the balloon deflates and they relax. Do this a few times. Your child is in the strong and powerful mountain pose.

Tree pose

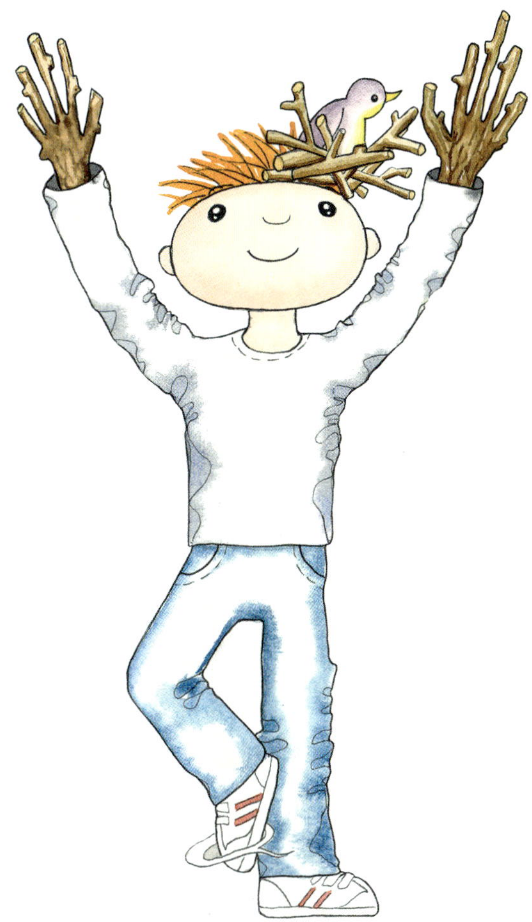

To become a Tree, ask your child to shift their weight over to one side and send roots down into the ground of the weighted foot. Next, ask them to focus on a spot in front of them that is not moving and then lift the other foot into tree posture. If their balance is a bit wobbly they can place their lifted foot simply on the other foot or they can place it onto the leg (ensuring their foot is not on the knee). Again in tree posture, ask them to notice how an inhalation expands their balloon lungs, and how the body relaxes with an exhalation. They can practice this wonderfully balancing pose several times on both sides.

Lion pose

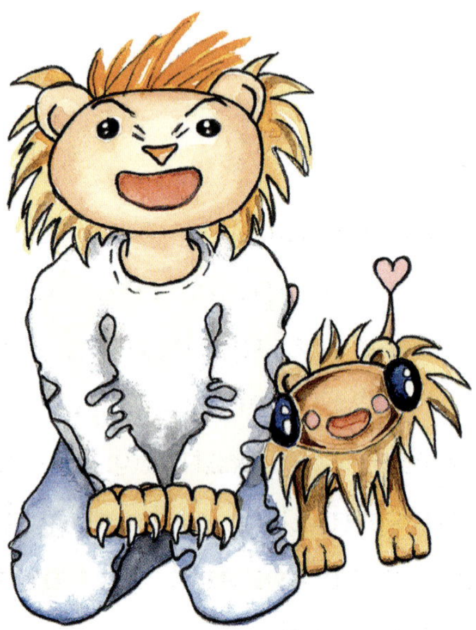

Ask your child to kneel with their feet touching behind them, and with the knees quite wide. Their hands should be placed flat on the floor in front of them. Encourage your child to scrunch up their face, move their mouth around and then stick their tongue out and make a breathless roar!

Face each other and do these roars together; be fearless lions and notice how this breathing is both empowering yet calming.

Cobra pose

From lion pose your child can slide onto their tummies and rest. Again ask them to notice their balloon lungs and to see whether they can still feel this lift on an inhalation, and how their body comes to rest on an exhalation. Even better, can they feel their tummies fill and empty, and the rise and fall this brings? This will promote abdominal breathing (known as proper breathing) which so many of us lose by adulthood.

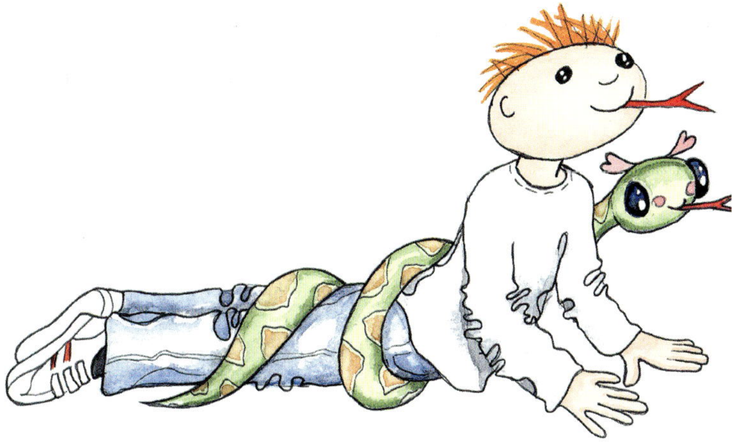

In cobra pose they place their hands flat on the ground next to their shoulders. With an inhalation the cobra uses the strength of their back to raise the upper part of their body. Then, as they place their body back to the ground, they can make a 'ssssss' noise as their lungs deflate. Making this sound is very therapeutic, as well as fun.

Dog pose

Start dog pose on all fours. Ask your child to straighten their legs and raise their bottoms up into the air. Ask them to feel the connection of their hands into the ground, and the soles of the feet coming down to the floor, and again to visualise strong roots from the feet growing deep into the ground. This is a lovely stretch for the back and really lengthens the back of the legs.

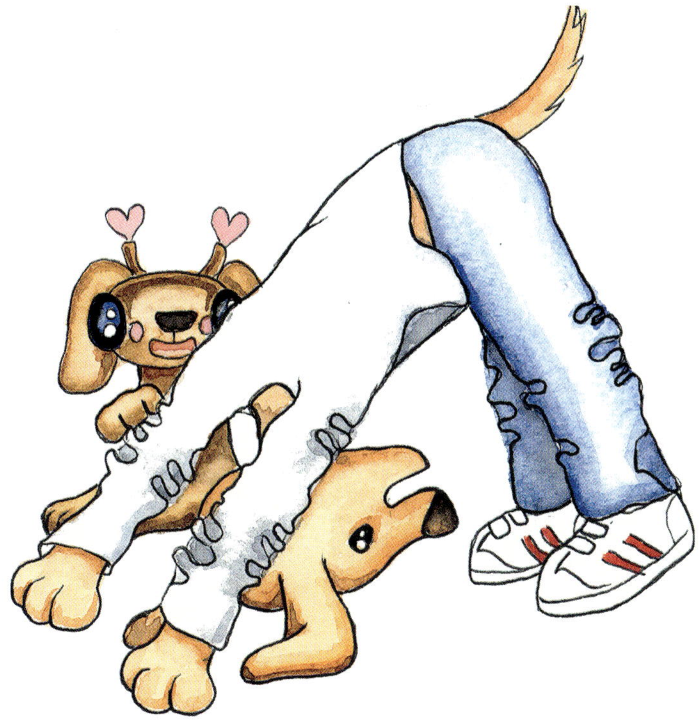

When your child is in the pose, ask them to wiggle their tail to allow more movement and mobility into the spine. Ask them how their balloon lungs feel up there. If they are holding their breath encourage them and remind them to keep breathing. Can they try and breathe into their tails? Again this will lengthen the breath and they may find their tails wiggle more!

Cat pose

Finally, encourage your child to use an exhalation to bring them down to all fours to practice cat pose.

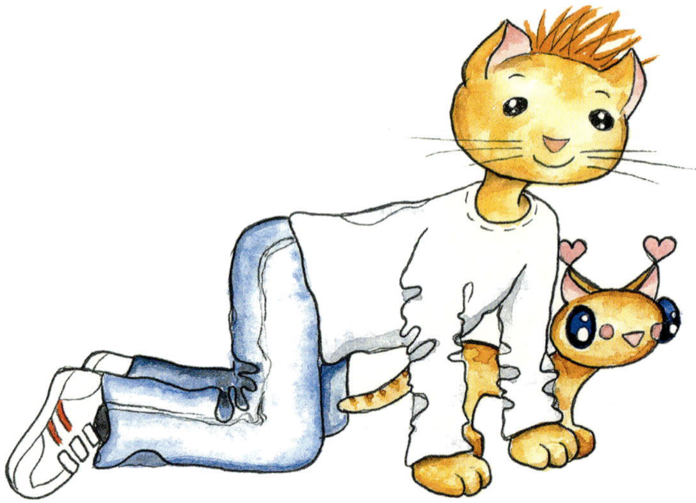

Play around with asking your child to feel like a cat, slinking around! Then with an inhalation ask the child to arch their back as much as they can, giving a good stretch, and then on an exhalation allow the back to concave. Don't get too hung up on the breath; the important thing is just to get your child moving in new ways.

This gives the whole spine a lovely stretch and moves your child into their body. Let them have lots of feline fun moving in and out of cat pose, and around the room.

Positive effects

These yoga postures help your child grow and maintain a strong and supple body and they also promote positive psychological effects. Mountain pose, for instance, can help your child stand their ground and increase confidence; tree pose focuses and calms the mind; lion pose is great for face and throat health and also increases concentration; cobra pose increases the flexibility of the back, removes stale air from the lungs and opens the heart; dog pose is a whole body stretch and strengthener; while cat pose is very calming and increases flexibility in the back. Remember to practice all the postures with your child and notice the positive effects within yourself!

Meditation and mindfulness

Buzzing-bee breath

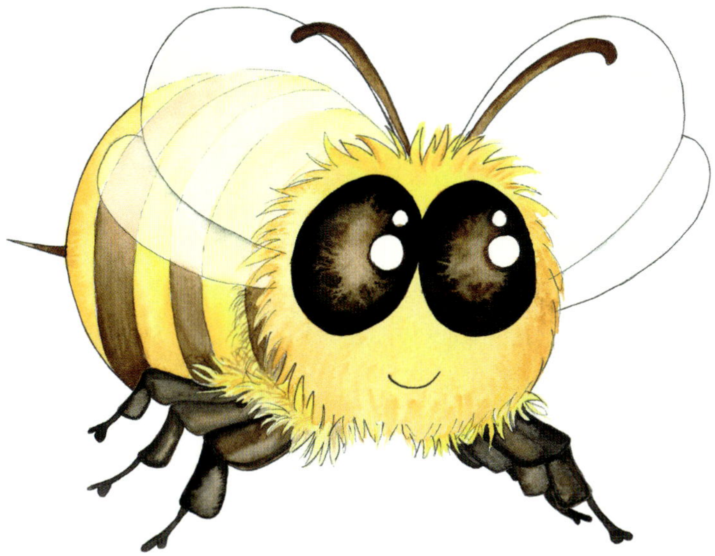

The buzzing-bee breath, is a really lovely way to introduce your child to meditation. It is incredibly calming and subtly directs your child's awareness into their inner world.

In terms of well-being, it is highly advantageous to come to know one's inner world. We tend to think of our world in terms of the physical, but we have a whole inner world populated by our thoughts and feelings. Coming to know our inner world, and to be aware of our mind and its tendencies, is therefore an important step in self-awareness.

This is particularly important in modern-day life, as the television and the Internet bombard our young with noise and images. Moreover, our heads are filled and reverberating with masses of information and trains of thought that lead our minds all over the place. How can we think clearly when our minds are so wild?

Mindfulness and meditation are becoming increasingly popular as they can teach us to listen to our thoughts with awareness and thus respond, rather than react. Given this, if our children can learn techniques to create peace and calm inside themselves it is an invaluable life skill and one highly associated with well-being. In the story, the inner world is referred to as the 'secret playground'. I can't emphasise how important the understanding and development of this 'secret playground' is for well-being throughout your child's life.

Prior to the 'buzzing-bee breath' exercise, it is useful to talk to your child about how the body literally 'talks' to them. Our body is ours for our whole life (so much comes and goes) and we must learn to look after it, respect it, and also learn to listen to it.

The body also holds a whole wealth of wisdom. Some simple examples of this are a rumbling tummy which is our body telling us it is hungry, or 'butterflies' fluttering in our tummies when we are nervous. Learning to listen to our bodies is a great skill to cultivate.

To begin the buzzing-bee breath, ask your child to kneel or sit cross legged, then put their lips together and go 'mmmm', for a whole exhalation. Ask them to go 'pp' as if they are letting the humming bee out of their mouth at the end of the exhalation. Then inhale and go again. Play with this buzzing noise and the sensations.

Super-sonic hearing

Next, ask your child to close their eyes and make quite a low humming noise. Tell them to listen really carefully when they stop humming (ask them to let the hum sound end naturally rather than adding the 'pp'). At the point when they stop humming they will be able to hear 'the furthest they have ever heard!' At this point the hearing accentuates and this is called 'super-sonic hearing' in the story. Ask them what they can hear. I have had some hilarious answers to this question!

Next, ask your child to repeat the humming breath and close their ears with their fingers. As the buzzing changes and internalises, ask them to try and feel it all around their body. Can they send the buzz down their feet, along their arms, up to the top of their head?

Using this technique should allow your child to begin to understand, visualise and come to know their 'secret playground'. In the longer term this helps to build their inner-confidence and self-awareness, and will serve as a valuable tool throughout their life.

Super-bright sight

Another technique contained in the story to increase mindfulness is known as 'super-bright sight', which helps your child to widen their awareness. This is important, as in the West our culture encourages us to think from the perspective of the individual, rather than the collective, and there is some evidence that this narrows our vision. Usually when we walk around we are not engaging our peripheral vision and we may even just be looking at the ground.

Recent psychological evidence indicates that noticing and appreciating the world around us (a type of gratitude) is one of the strongest indicators of well-being. To rephrase this, it is evident that simply slowing down and taking the time to notice and appreciate what is going on in the present moment is really good for you. I often think how incredible it is that such simplicity can have such a profound effect on our well-being, yet the techniques to cultivate this are not widely known or practiced…madness!

It is worth practicing 'super-bright sight' a few times so that you can confidently explain it to your child. Stretch your arms out in front of you with your index fingers pointing up to the ceiling.

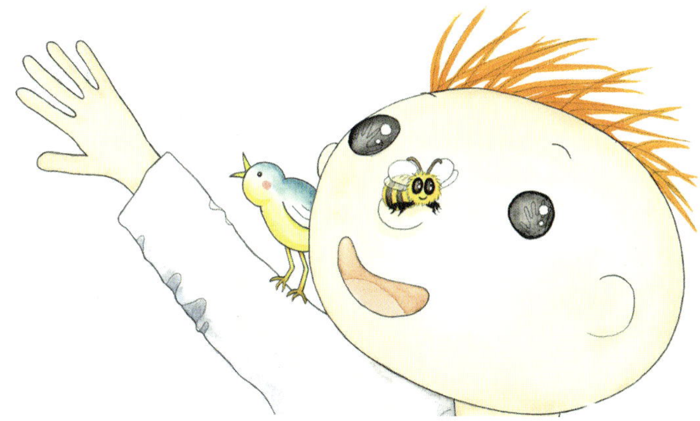

Next, keep your focus in front of you and then move your hands to the side (focus still in front). Find the point where you are still looking ahead but you can still see your fingers in your peripheral vision.

Keep this awareness and focus and drop your arms. You will notice that your eyes, awareness and focus feel different. In yoga they consider that it may even be harder to think and stress when this 'super-bright sight' is engaged. Just imagine how useful this is to develop!

Teach the technique to your child and then go somewhere safe in the garden, or in a park, and walk around with the 'super-bright sight' engaged. Notice how much you see, like an animal your vision and awareness becomes more instinctual. You can have loads of fun with this and it's really quite fascinating.

Looking after each other

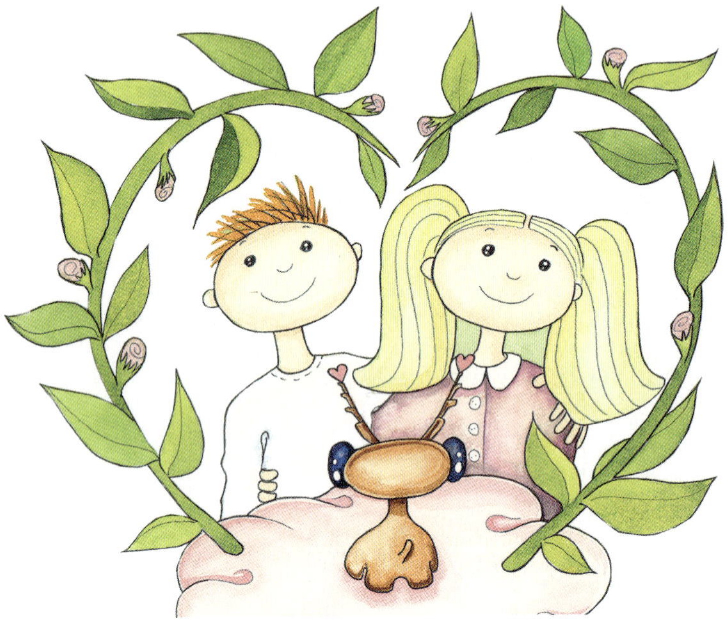

Most parents will teach the importance of co-operation and working together, and being kind to one another. Yoga/meditation-based techniques can encourage this and, although not well known, these work particularly well with young children.

I will explain one such technique that I have found to have a wonderfully positive and gentle effect on children. This is based on the Buddhist loving-kindness meditation.

Begin with the buzzing-bee breath and work with this until your child settles down. Next, ask your child to close their eyes and think of someone that they love who is smiling at them.

This is fun to do as your child will start to smile as they think of this smiling person. Ask them where this feeling of love arises in their body, and also ask them to describe its colour (again this is an excellent way of encouraging your child to come to know their inner world of feelings and emotions).

Next, ask your child to paint their whole body with this colour and to then think of a friend and paint this friend with the same colour. You can also ask them to paint one of their teachers with the colour, or encourage them to paint lots of people, or even to paint the whole world.

I do this with my children quite often and afterwards they are so gentle, happy and calm. I reflect with them on how lovely it is to send positive feeling to people, which is like sending gifts to people without them even knowing! For younger children you can call this 'heart power' or 'super-magic love' and get them to take this out of their body and sprinkle it everywhere they go.

I find this useful in teaching children how their inner worlds can affect the external world. It also helps encourage pro-social behaviour, gratitude and emotional intelligence, and it is delightful for your child to explore being led by the heart rather than the head.

Looking after nature and the environment

There has been recent interest in nature-deficit disorder, and worrying statistics about the lack of outdoor play and its links to obesity and mental-health problems. However, opportunities for learning about the environment are increasing, as seen by the popularity of forest and wood schools and also by campaigns by conservation charities, such as the National Trust.

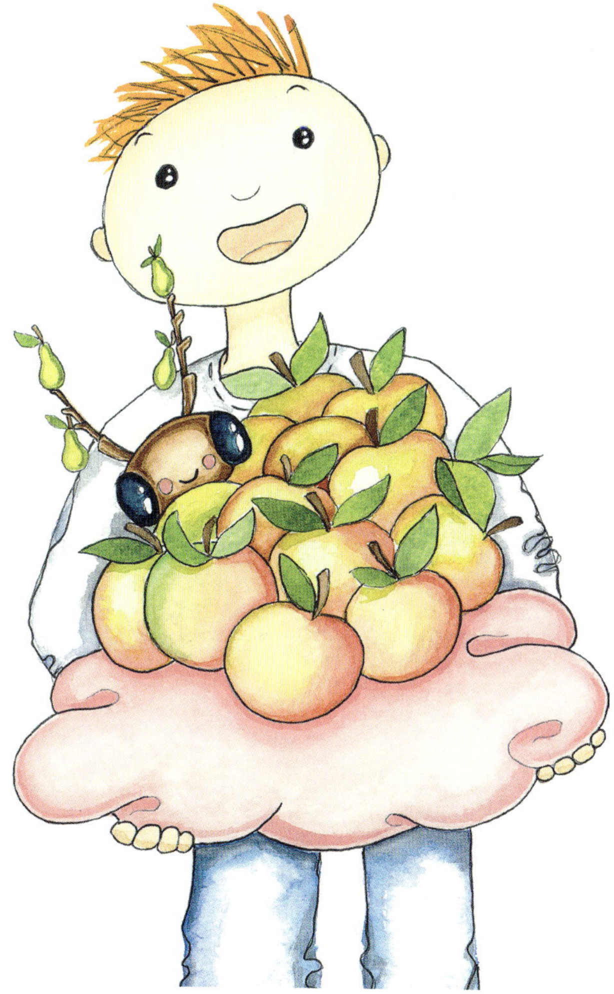

What I feel would be useful to explore is how we can teach interconnectedness through nature and the breath. I have done this work in schools and with my own children, and it is a wonderful opportunity to introduce children to deeper topics.

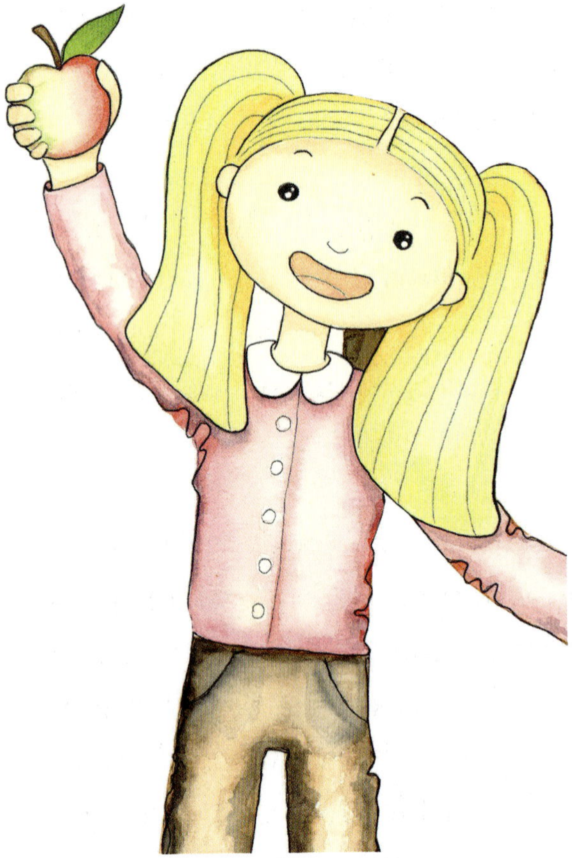

Building on the earlier exercises, and encouraging your child's awareness of the breath, we can talk to our children about how the breath carries life. For instance, if we breathe deeply our breath takes more oxygen to the body and fills it with life and energy.

It is also useful to consider life directly through nature. For example, in a recent workshop I took some leaves into class and we reflected upon their veins. We placed the leaf on our hands and talked about how life runs through the leaf and also through other plants and animals, as well as us. We also talked a little about what happens when life leaves the leaf and we passed around a leaf that had become all crispy and brown. Finally, we talked of how we can cultivate life and encourage it to grow and thrive, both in nature and also within ourselves, through keeping healthy and strong both mentally and physically.

These topics allow us to acknowledge, celebrate and give thanks for nature and life. I find that if our children respect all forms of life (human, animal and plant) and feel that we are all part of this same experience, they naturally become more sensitive and responsive to nature.

I have found these types of discussions, even with quite young children, to be very comforting and awe-inspiring. I also feel for children to sense this interconnection instils a deep sense of belonging that is somewhat profound.

Celebrating life and inspiring awe in our children

Recent research on children's well-being suggests that children are the most self-absorbed and competitive in recent history. Although the causes of this are debatable, research also suggests that inspiring awe is a wonderful antidote.

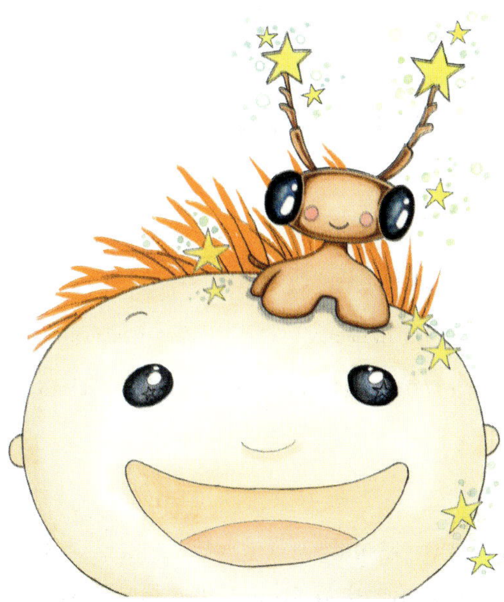

Awe is the experience, or recognition, of something larger and bigger than the self. For example, standing at the foot of an imposing mountain, looking out to the ocean, or considering the wonders of the solar system, can all create feelings of awe.

Academic research suggests that self absorption and narcissism is on the increase in young people. However, the emotion of awe can help balance the preconception that we are the centre of the world.

When we notice and appreciate the world around us (don't forget this is a type of gratitude) we become mindful of its greatness and all of a sudden we can feel quite small, yet part of this great whole. We can behold the great paradox of life and, as if by magic, all the little things in our life, the niggles that seemed so big, can disappear. This wider perspective (being inspired by awe) can for that moment, make us realise how precious our life is and this can be a great motivating force.

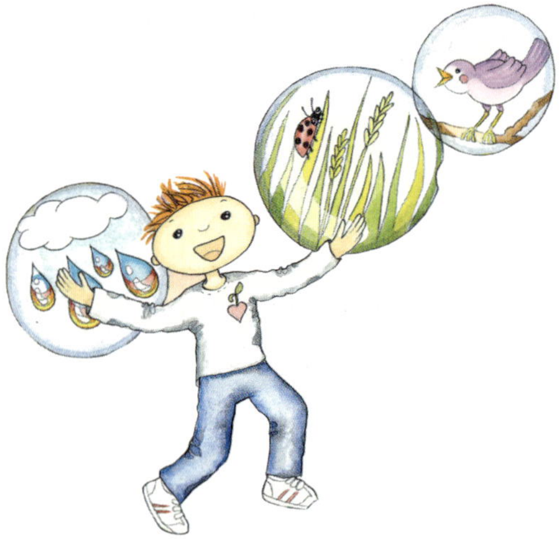

I believe these feelings to be hugely beneficial for both our children's and our planet's well-being.

It is really exciting to talk to our children about their wildest dreams, inspire them to realise that anything is possible. When we start noticing the world around us, and the worlds within us, it is truly inspiring, and there are no limits. I love tempting and exciting children (and adults) with the last line from Mary Oliver's poem *The Summer Day*...'Tell me, what is it you plan to do with your one wild and precious life?

The enchanted child project

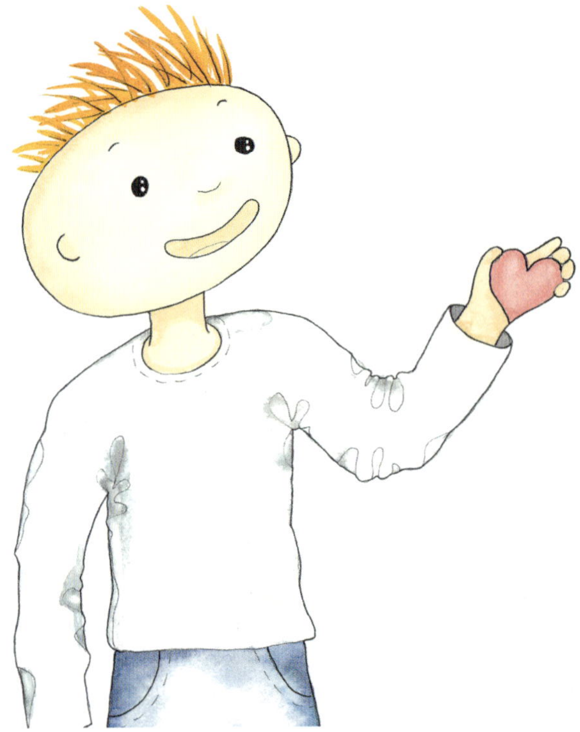

This book forms the basis of *The Enchanted Child Project*, which I started two years ago. The project's vision is in a way my own wildest dream, one that is driven by a desire for a better way of living and a better way of being. Growing this project, nurturing children and connecting with like-minded adults is part of what I would like to do with my one wild and precious life.

In starting *The Enchanted Child Project* I began to notice and appreciate more and more the amazing world that we live in. I also began to realise the complexity, yet simplicity, of the body and the mind, and of the human condition.

It has changed my life in a tremendously positive way, and has helped me greatly in being a parent and trying to share this vision with my children. In many of the realms I work in, I'm noticing more and more that times are changing. It is very exciting that the modern-day psychology research is converging with ancient wisdom and an alternative path to well-being is unfolding. This book is an attempt to raise awareness of, and to support, nourish and cultivate this path.

I believe there to be an inherent beauty in this approach, and certainly when I began on this journey it was a trail of positive occurrences. I found people, not just parents, on the same journey and many have supported and joined me.

I started to notice and appreciate those around me, and in my community. From this I found great talent, a local artist who illustrated this book, a dancer, a graphic designer and musician, who helped me turn the book into a school's programme.

Most importantly, however, it reminded me of how our children—my children and your children—are little sparks of creativity and wonder just waiting to blossom. It is therefore truly a joy to nourish and nurture our children's roots so they can grow strong and bloom in the most spectacular way.

I wrote this book with so much love and I hope it will be an encouragement for you and your child to embark (hand-in-hand) on this path, or act as an inspiration for those of you already on your way. One thing I am sure of, and I am also delighted to confirm, is that this journey is one filled with life, love, excitement, colour, awe, inspiration and light...how wonderful!

Jeannine Goh March 2014

The Enchanted Gallery

There is something about a child's imagination and their connection to wonder that is truly amazing. Their capacity to dream can be wild and it possesses no boundaries, and no constraints. Children are also our inspiration and so often our teachers. We may be there to guide and nourish them, but in exchange they enchant, delight and excite us, and they can whisk us off to magical places that we as adults have now forgotten.

In celebration of our children's creativity and their inherent capacity for love, awe and wonder, I thought it would be wonderful to end this book with a gallery of children's work. The brief was simple, after exploring the story (with the help of the parent's guidance) the children were asked to simply draw whatever they liked.

We would like to open this gallery to all children who engage with this book. If your child is inspired to create we would love to hear from you. They might draw a picture, write a poem, or may even create something we had never imagined!

Please send all creations to inspire@awespace.org. Some of these will appear on our website and some will be published in the Enchanted Gallery at the end of the next edition of this book!

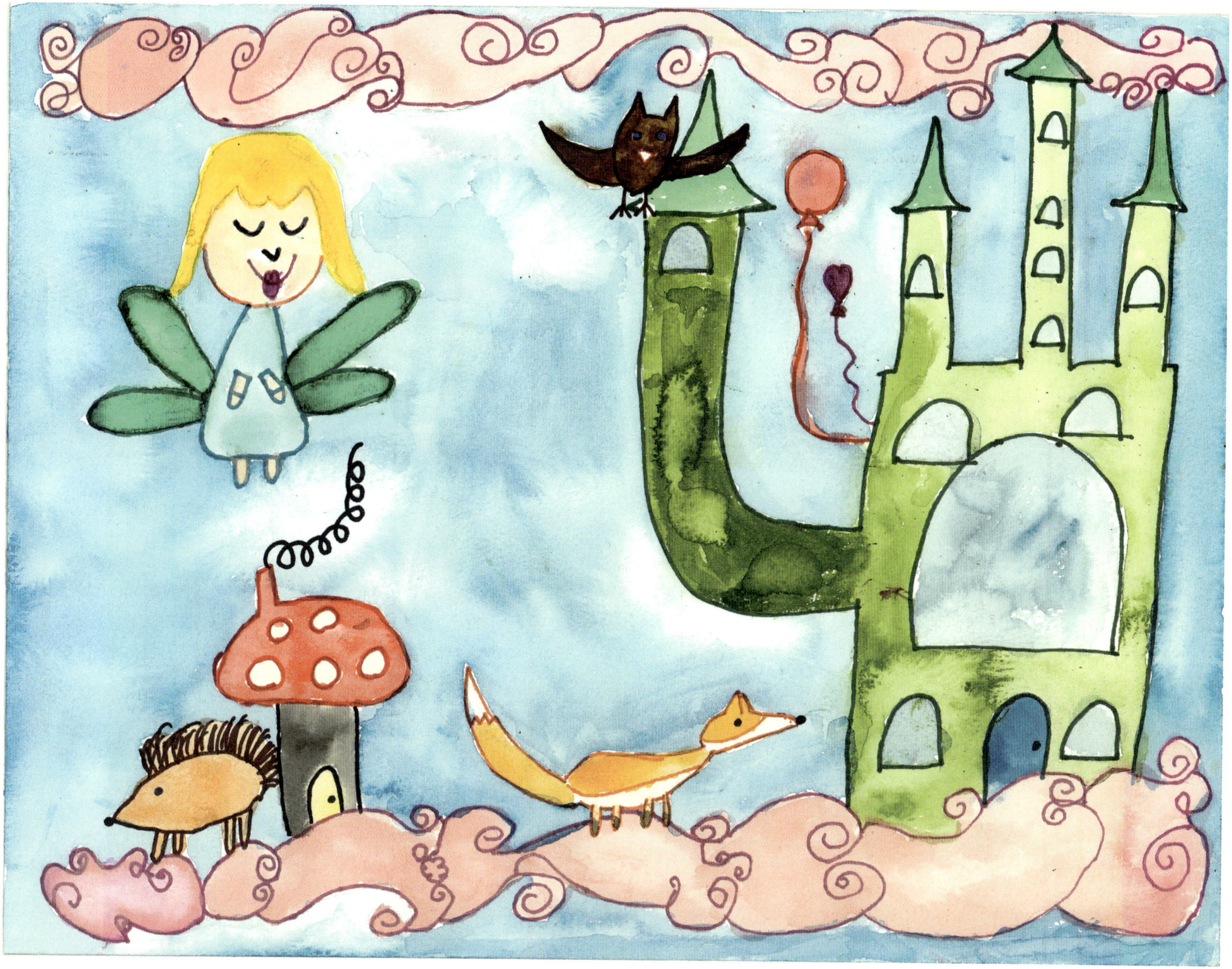

Ruby Owen Hull aged 7

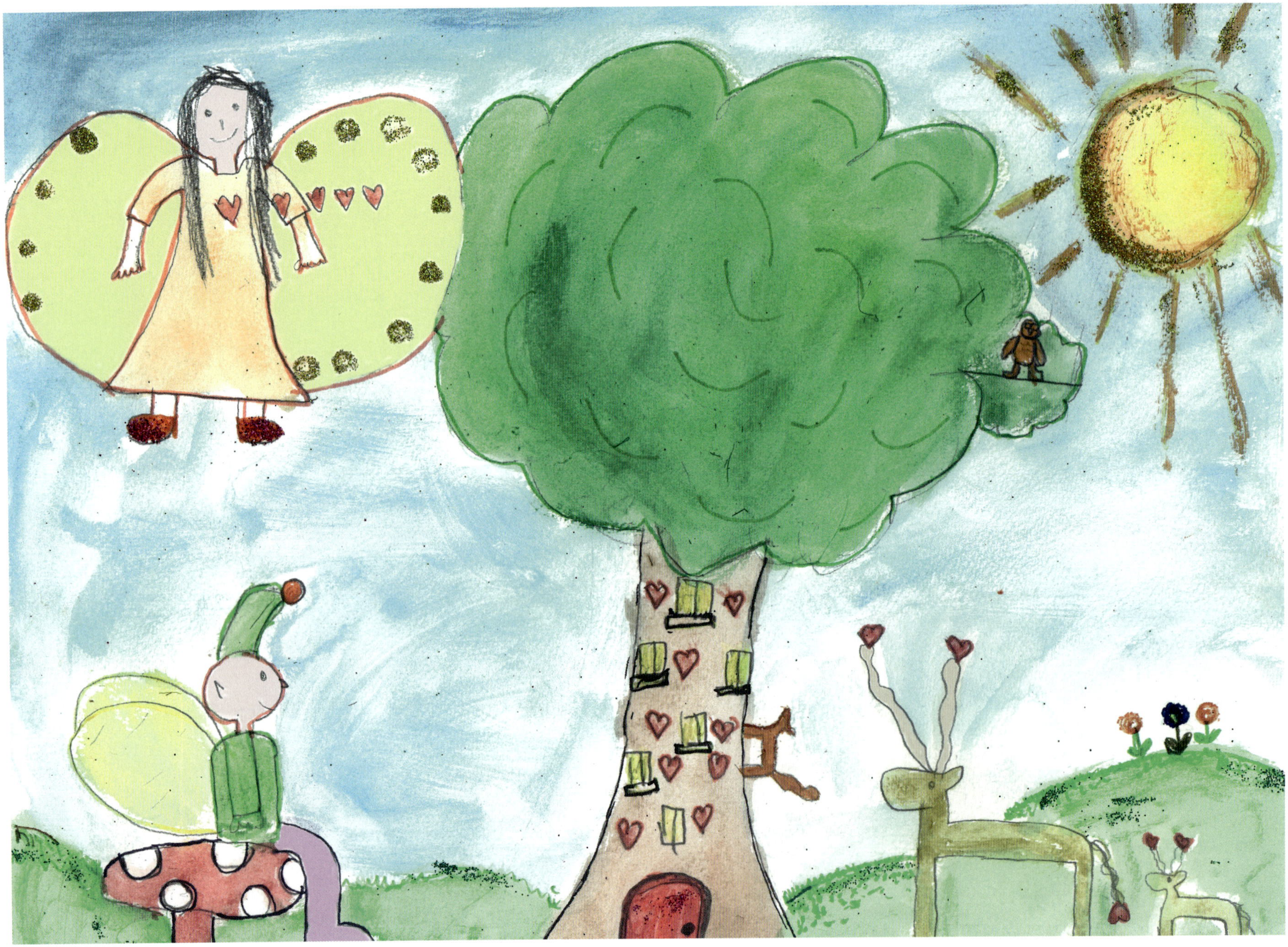

Jasmine Gregory aged 6

Can you draw?

What can you detect with your super-sonic hearing?

What can you spot with your super-bright sight?

What is your wildest dream?

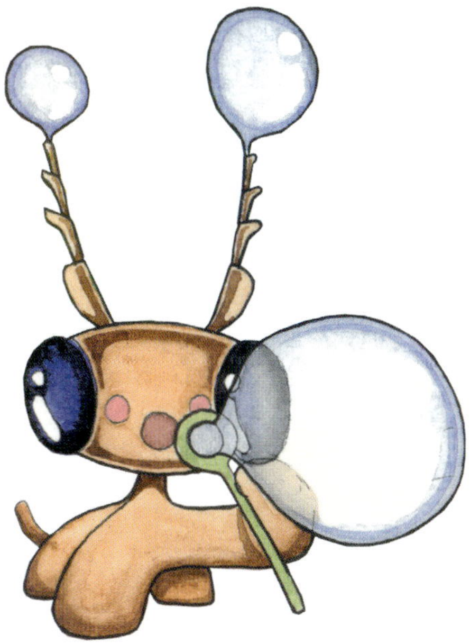

Did you know?

The worrying news

A 2014 report by the Royal Society of Arts suggests that 'the requirement of schools to develop the broader human qualities of their pupils has become side-lined due to the overwhelming pressure placed on them to deliver better exam results'.

A UNICEF study placed the UK at the bottom of the child well-being league tables among developed countries.

A recent academic study indicates that young people are self-absorbed and the most self-concerned and competitive in recent history.

Research indicates that our children are becoming more disconnected with nature which can lead to a physical and mental illness termed nature-deficit disorder.

Did you know?

The good news

Academic research indicates that a simple process of giving thanks increases well-being.

A UNESCO-endorsed initiative suggests that global citizenship and tolerance can be stimulated by considering the vastness and beauty of the Universe, and our place within it.

A recent study indicates that mindfulness interventions have a positive impact on stress and are attractive to schools and educators.

After just ten days there is significant enhancement in well-being, and in particular happiness, achievement and interpersonal relationships, through the practice of yoga.

The Enchanted Child Project

The Enchanted Child Project is a not-for-profit organisation with charitable aims that has been funded by UnLtd, The National Lottery and The Royal Society of Arts for our pioneering work in children's well-being. We are a social enterprise and the profits from this book are returned to the project to continue our good work. By buying this book you are helping us to engage with more families, schools and children to create positive change.

In addition to this book, we also produce our own magical and magnificent music. We noticed that there is a lack of musically intelligent songs for children that have strong and positive messages. We have therefore created a series of songs to compliment this book that explore the body and mind, friendship and community, and nature and awe. With the help of some extremely talented producers we have created some fantastic music of varying styles and genres. This is strong and inspiring music that appeals to both children and adults; a wonderful shared experience for families. You can download a sample and find out how to buy the CD at http://www.awespace.org

We also run a Soulful School programme. We have collaborated with drama practitioners, musicians, and dance/creative-movement practitioners to bring the Enchanted Child story to life. In a series of workshops, the children recreate Ted's journey and they become the protagonists of the story. Our passionate and vibrant practitioners inspire the children to dance, sing and dramatise the story, and this is skilfully balanced with moments of deep silence and contemplation of life-lessons. Our Soulful School programme culminates in a performance of the story that incorporates our songs and dialogue from the children. A fantastic celebration of who we are, and of life!

For more information about our school programme
visit http://www.awespace.org

The Enchanted Child

Awespace

This book is published by Awespace. Awespace is a not-for-profit organisation, with charitable aims, which has a clear vision of a healthy, happy future for all.

Awespace creates a space to consider what is important in life; a place for you, your children, your family, our schools and our communities to find inspiration for a better way of living or a better way of being.

At Awespace we recognise the desperate need for more space in our lives. Awe is an emotion that we experience when we have a sense of something greater and bigger than ourselves. Our perception and awareness expands ad infinitum. We believe there to be a great freedom in this moment. We can reflect the greatness of the world with our own meagreness. In this moment our worries become insignificant and our life's possibilities endless. We call this Awespace, a precious expansive place in our minds that we can all develop. When Awespace is created within the mind, when all the clutter and chatter is removed, creativity and wisdom are free to flow and everything and anything are possible.

Our website provides a virtual space with inspiring information and resources; a place where we can gather and contemplate.

Visit us and join us in creating positive change

http://www.awespace.org

AWESPACE

About the author

Jeannine is a doctor of psychology, lecturer, yoga practitioner, author and singer song-writer. She is deeply committed to children's well-being and to considering how we can create better ways of living and better ways of being. She lives in Manchester with her husband and two beautiful children where she can be found conspiring to bring creativity and colour into anything looking a bit grey.

About the illustrator

Sam is a professional artist who has exhibited in the UK and internationally. She is at her very happiest when she is drawing, painting or otherwise making an idea come to life, whilst listening to music and sipping tea. Sam lives in Manchester with her family.

Ted is bored. But then his world changes forever when he has a visit from Omu the Wise. Whisked away on a fast-paced adventure, he discovers his hidden inner powers, helps a friend in distress, finds magic in nature and then has a super-fantastic party!

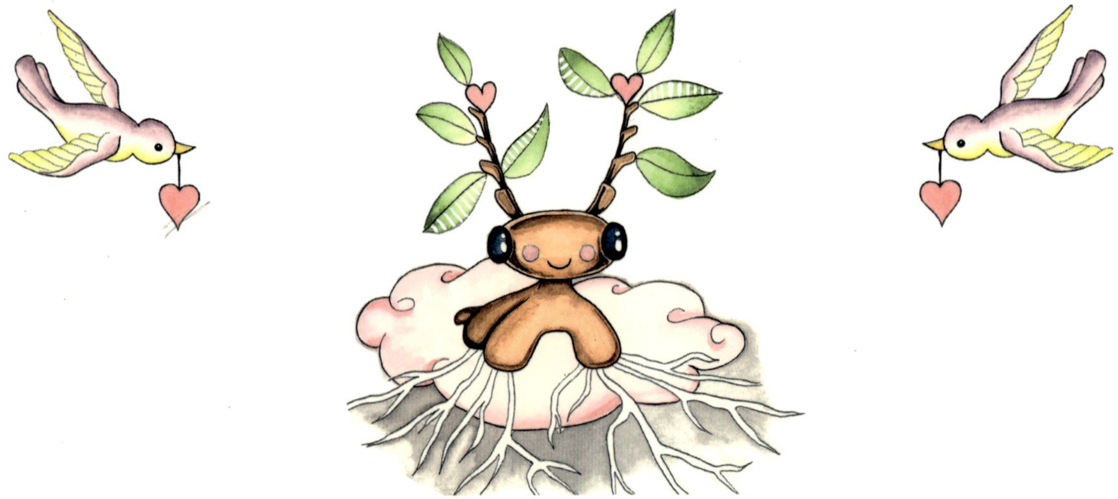

This uplifting children's story is a spark for exploring and encouraging deeper connections with the body and mind, friends and community, nature, the wider-world and the cosmos. Combining ancient wisdom with modern-day psychology, the story playfully engages your child in various techniques (including yoga, mindfulness and meditation) known to have wonderfully positive effects. This is complimented by a lovingly written and skilfully created parent's guide to developing these techniques, and for exploring some of life's bigger questions. A beautifully illustrated book and an amazing adventure to embark on!

AWESPACE

£7.99

ISBN 978-0-9929095-0-5

00799

9 780992 909505